COMMON BILE DUCT EXPLORATION

DEVELOPMENTS IN SURGERY

J.M. Greep, H.A.J. Lemmens, D.B. Roos, H.C. Urschel, eds., Pain in Shoulder and Arm: An Integrated View
ISBN 90 247 2146 6

B. Niederle, Surgery of the Biliary Tract
ISBN 90 247 2402 3

J.A. Nakhosteen & W. Maassen, eds., Bronchology: Research, Diagnostic and Therapeutic Aspects
ISBN 90 247 2449 X

R. van Schilfgaarde, J.C. Stanley, P. van Brummelen & E.H. Overbosch, eds., Clinical Aspects of Renovascular Hypertension
ISBN 0 89838 574 1

G.M. Abouna, ed. & A.G. White, ass. ed., Current Status of Clinical Organ Transplantation. With some Recent Developments in Renal Surgery
ISBN 0 89838 635 7

A. Cuschieri & G. Berci, Common Bile Duct Exploration
ISBN 0 89838 639 X

A. Cuschieri & G. Berci, Common Bile Duct Exploration in combination with video tape, Operative and Postoperative Biliary Endoscopy
ISBN 0 89838 692 6

COMMON BILE DUCT EXPLORATION

Intraoperative investigations in biliary tract surgery

by

Professor A. CUSCHIERI, MD, ChM, FRCS (Eng), FRCS (Ed)
Professor and Head of Department of Surgery, Ninewells Hospital and Medical School
University of Dundee, Dundee, Scotland
Consultant Surgeon to the Tayside Health Board

G. BERCI, MD, FACS
Associate Director of Surgery, Cedars-Sinai Medical Center
and Clinical Professor of Surgery, UCLA School of Medicine

With contributions from

J.A. HAMLIN, MD
Staff Radiologist, Chief, Section of G.I. Radiology
Cedars-Sinai Medical Center, Los Angeles, USA

MARGARET PAZ-PARTLOW, MA, MFA
Research Assistant, Section of Surgical Endoscopy
Department of Surgery
Cedars-Sinai Medical Center, Los Angeles, USA

1984 **MARTINUS NIJHOFF PUBLISHERS**
a member of the KLUWER ACADEMIC PUBLISHERS GROUP
BOSTON / DORDRECHT / LANCASTER

Distributors

for the United States and Canada: Kluwer Academic Publishers, 190 Old Derby Street, Hingham, MA 02043, USA

for the UK and Ireland: Kluwer Academic Publishers, MTP Press Limited, Falcon House, Queen Square, Lancaster LA1 1RN, England

for all other countries: Kluwer Academic Publishers Group, Distribution Center, P.O. Box 322, 3300 AH Dordrecht, The Netherlands

Library of Congress Cataloging in Publication Data

```
Cuschieri, Alfred.
   Common bile duct exploration.

   (Developments in surgery)
   Includes index.
   1. Bile-ducts--Surgery.  I. Berci, George, 1921-
II. Title.  III. Series.  [DNLM: 1. Cholangiography--
Handbooks.  2. Biliary tract diseases--Surgery--Hand-
books.  3. Surgery, Operative--Handbooks. W1 DE8S
W1 39 C984c]
RD546.C87 1984      617'.556      84-1614
```

ISBN 978-94-009-6005-3   ISBN 978-94-009-6003-9 (eBook)

DOI 10.1007/978-94-009-6003-9

Copyright

CONTENTS

1. Introduction   1

2. Review of existing problems in biliary tract surgery   3

3. Surgical approach and principles   7
   1. Introduction   7
   2. Prophylactic measures   7
   2.1. Infectious complications   7
   2.2. Haemorrhagic complications   8
   2.3. Renal failure   8
   3. Pre-operative biliary decompression in the jaundiced patient   9
   4. Operative principles   9
   4.1. Surgical access   9
   4.2. Patient positioning   9
   4.3. Appropriate incision   9
   4.4. Illumination of the operating field   10
   4.5. Packing   10
   4.6. Exposure of relevant anatomy   10
   5. Drainage of the supracolic compartment after biliary operations   11

4. Operative cholangiography (*in cooperation with J.A. Hamlin and M. Paz-Partlow*)   19
   1. Introduction   10
   2. Common bile duct explorations   00
   3. Unsuspected stones   20
   4. Cannulation techniques   20
   5. Initial and/or completion cholangiograms   20
   6. Standard technique   21
   6.1. Technique and equipment   21
   6.2. Patient's positioning   20
   6.3. Scout film   22
   6.4. Injected volume   22
   6.5. Contrast material   22
   6.6. Coordination of exposure   22
   6.7. Mobile C-arm fluoroscope   22
   7. Fluoro-cholangiography   22
   7.1. Easy positioning of the patient   23
   7.2. Optimal beam collimation   23
   7.3. Shorter exposure time   23
   7.4. Automatic exposure control   23

7.5.	Minimal technician activity	23
7.6.	Control of the exposure sequence	23
7.7.	Serial films	23
7.8.	Decreased examination time	24
7.9.	Indirect radiography	24
8.	Anomalies of surgical importance	24
8.1.	Short cystic duct	24
8.2.	Drainage of cystic duct in the right hepatic duct	24
8.3.	Aberrant ducts	24
8.4.	Ductal diverticula and choledochocele	24
8.5.	The acute or emergency case	24
9.	General aspects	25
10.	Radiation protection	25
11.	The cystic duct	25
12.	Cholecysto-cholangiogram	25
13.	The choledocho-cholangiogram	26
13.1.	Direct needle puncture	26
13.2.	Butterfly needle puncture	26
13.3.	Special needle clamp	26
13.4.	T-tube insertion	26
14.	Contact selective cholangiography	27
15.	Reason for failure for operative cholangiography	27
15.1.	Overfilled ducts	27
15.2.	Underfilled ducts	27
15.3.	Poor quality films	27
15.4.	Improper positioning	27
15.5.	Obscured field	27
16.	Artifacts	28
17.	Complications of operative cholangiography	28
18.	Reformed calculi	28
19.	Complications of T-tube removal in the post-operative period	28
20.	Results of operative cholangiography	30
20.1.	Advantages	30
20.2.	Disadvantages	30
5.	Operative biliary endoscopy (cholangioscopy) (*in cooperation with M. Paz-Partlow*)	55
1.	Introduction	55
2.	Instrumentation	55
2.1.	Accessories	56
3.	Technique	56
3.1.	Mobilization of the duodenum	56
3.2.	Endoscopic appearance	57
3.3.	The cystic stump remnant	57
4.	Endoscopic anatomy and pathology	57
4.1.	Normal findings	57
4.2.	Cholangitis	57
4.3.	Calculi	57
4.4.	Ampullary stenosis	58
4.5.	Neoplasms	58

4.6. Miscellaneous   58
5.   Repeated cholangioscopy   58
6.   Complications   59
7.   General aspects   59
7.1. Sterilization   59
7.2. Maintenance   59
8.   Evaluation of results   59
9.   Conclusions   59

6.   Biliary manometry and debimetry   71
     1.   Introduction   71
     2.   Usage   71
     3.   Pharmacolgy of the sphincter of Oddi (SO)   71
     3.1. Effect of hormones and peptides   71
     3.2. Effect of pharmacological agents   72
     4.   Biliary pressure indices   72
     4.1. Resting (initial, interdigestive) pressure   72
     4.2. Passage (yield, opening) pressure   72
     4.3. Filling pressure curves   72
     4.4. Residual pressure   73
     4.5. Flow rate (debimetry)   73
     4.6. Incremental pressure and recovery time   73
     5.   Dynamic (transducer) manometry   73
     5.1. Endoscopic sphincter zone activity   73
     5.2. Technique of operative biliary manometry   73
     6.   Disorders of the sphincter of Oddi   74
     6.1. Iatrogenic stricture   74
     6.2. Papillitis/Oedema   74
     6.3. Papillary stenosis (choledocho-duodenal junctional stenosis)   75
     6.4. Functional disorders   75

7.   Exploration of the common bile duct   81
     1.   Introduction   81
     2.   Technique of CBD exploration   81
     2.1. Mobilization of duodenum and head of pancreas   81
     2.2. Exposure of the CBD   81
     2.3. Choledochotomy   82
     2.4. Cholangioscopy   82
     2.5. Additional procedures   82
     2.6. Insertion of T-tube   82
     2.7. Closure of choledochotomy wound   83
     3.   Trans-duodenal exploration od CBD   83
     4.   Intra-hepatic calculi   83
     5.   Assessment of terminal end of the CBD and sphincteric region   84
     6.   Post-operative removal of T-tube   84
     7.   Conclusion   84

8.   Postoperative removal of retained stones through the T-Tube tract (*in cooperation with J.A. Hamlin*)   89

VIII

1. Introduction   89
2. Stone extraction via the T-tube   89
3. Endoscopic method   89
4. Preparation for stone extraction   90
5. Technique   90
6. Results   91
7. Complications   91
8. Discussion   91

Index of Subjects   99

CHAPTER 1

INTRODUCTION

This book was conceived as a descriptive atlas of routine biliary surgery i.e., cholecystectomy and exploration of the common bile duct. For the project the two authors worked together for one week at Ninewells Hospital and Medical School, Dundee on a series of patients with biliary tract disease especially selected for the exercise. With the consent of the Tayside Health Board and the patients concerned, all the operations and peri-operative procedures were filmed by the photographic members of the team, Mr. and Mrs. Paz-Partlow. Additional case material has been obtained from Cedars Sinai Medical Center, Los Angeles.

The aim of the monograph has been to produce a practical manual to serve as a road map to operative technique and decision making during billiary tract surgery. We have incorporated throughout the book practical hints which we have found from experience to be useful and pertinent to expeditious biliary surgery.

The second objective of the monograph has been to emphasize prophylactic measures against peri-operative complications and operative injuries to the biliary tract since a large cohort of complications, serious or otherwise, following biliary tract surgery is largely preventable with careful planning, correct intra-operative decision making and safe and meticulous surgical technique.

Biliary surgical practice has evolved particularly in the last two decades. The surgeon has now at his disposal certain intra-operative investigations such as cholangiography and cholangioscopy which indicate the precise pathological anatomy and therefore the right operative procedure in addition to ensuring against missed pathology. Adequate training and familiarity with these procedures are essential to their reliability. Operative cholangiography should be performed routinely. It adds little to the operating time and provides the most reliable indication for common bile duct exploration. The cholangioscope allows a *visual* exploration of the biliary tree and permits the removal of common bile duct calculi and other procedures such as biopsy under direct visual control. Both procedures have been described in detail with emphasis on the practical aspects of their use. The era of blind bilary surgery is over and the sooner this message is received by all concerned, the better the outcome of biliary surgical practice overall.

It has not been our intention to produce a comprehensive reference textbook of biliary tract sugery. We hope, however, that we have achieved the objectives listed above and trust that this monograph will be found useful especially by our less experienced surgical colleagues. Although the well informed surgeon is not necessarily a safe one, the misinformed is a definite liability. Our training programmes should be aimed at producing skillful surgical operators well versed in the intraoperative investigational techniques and equipped with up-to-date information on surgical disorders. The theoretical and practical aspects of surgical training go hand in hand. This monograph represents such a mix. We have tried to reflect the general consensus of opinion over controversial matters and trust that the account is an objective one. It is difficult, however, to write such a book without incorporating individual practical hints born of experience and audit and for this we make no apologies since we know them to be useful.

Acknowledgements

In the first instance we are indebted to the patients at Ninewells Hospital and Medical School who so readily agreed to have their operation filmed and to

2

the Tayside Health Board for official approval to go ahead with the project. Excellent technical help was provided by Mr. M. Ettle (Chief Technician) during the filming.

We are thankful to the surgical staff members of the Department of Surgery CSMC for their collaboration, to Dr. J. Yadegar and Dr. S. Shapiro (Ch. 4 case 2) for allowing us to present these cases.

We would like to thank Karl Storz Co., Ltd, for the financial support in relation to expenditure incurred by Dr. Berci and his photographic team on the occasion of their visit to Ninewells. His generous grant enabled us to make the companion film "Operative and Post-Operative Biliary Endoscopy". (This film is available from the publisher, as a video tape.) We are also grateful to Mr. and Mrs. Paz-Partlow for their photographic and art work, especially to Mrs. M. Paz-Partlow who made the drawing on the cover. The illustrations to the various chapters were ably undertaken by Miss M. Sneddon (Ninewells Hospital and Medical School, Dundee) and Mrs. M. De Bose (Cedars Sinai Medical Center). We are indebted to our secretaries Mrs. J. Mackenzie and Ms. A. Wasser who prepared the manuscript with great efficiency and style. Finally we are grateful to the publishers for their advice, guidance, patience and for implementing our ideas on the layout as far as was practically possible.

A. Cuschieri
G. Berci

CHAPTER 2

REVIEW OF EXISTING PROBLEMS IN BILIARY TRACT SURGERY

Cholecystectomy is the most frequently performed abdominal surgical operation. Although the overall reported mortality is low, estimated at 2–3%, the morbidity in terms of residual stones, unnecessary CBD explorations, bile duct injuries and infective complications remains considerable.

There are no reliable figures for the percentage of patients who require secondary intervention following cholecystectomy. It is true that nowadays endoscopic techniques for removal of residual stones materially reduce the number of secondary surgical interventions for this complication. Nevertheless there remains a hard core of patients who require further surgery, often necessitating transfer to an institution where special expertise is available for dealing with secondary and tertiary biliary operations.

The extent of the problem can be summarized by reference to the number of cholecystectomies performed in the U.S.A. This averages 3500 per 10^6 inhabitants per annum (735 000). Some 20% of these patients (150 000) will also undergo CBD explorations which will be negative in 20% (30 000). The expected overall incidence of retained stones related to the total number of cholecystectomies is 10% (73 500). This is almost certainly a gross underestimate since the figures are obtained from patients undergoing postoperative T-tube cholangiography, whereas some 80% of patients cannot be checked postoperatively since they do not have a T-tube. If the residual stone rate is related to only those patients who have undergone CBD exploration with insertion of a T-tube, the available evidence suggests a residual stone rate of 10 to 20%. Even if the majority of these patients (90%) can be successfully treated by endoscopic extraction through the T-tube tract, the cost overall to any Health Care System whether private or public is considerable, as is the loss of earned income and hours of man work of these unfortunate patients. Some 13% will still require a further operation at the end of the day and this will usually entail a bilio-digestive by-pass procedure. The socio-economic impact on this subgroup is considerable and often results in costly litigation. Residual stones at best delay recovery and return to gainful employment by 6 weeks. Of course some patients never make it, dying as they do of cholangitis and septicaemia or of a cardiovascular complication particularly if they are above 60 years of age. In any event both the morbidity and mortality following secondary biliary intervention for residual calculous disease are significantly higher than after primary biliary surgery.

Infective complications after biliary tract surgery are usually due to aerobic gram-negative coliforms although serious anaerobic infections do occur. Prophylactic short term antibiotic therapy with a cephalosporin will markedly reduce the infective complication rate and is indicated in patients who are at risk. The high risk factors have been identified and include jaundice, recent rigors and pyrexia, emergency operation, old age, previous surgery on the billiary tract, CBD obstruction and stones in the common duct.

Undoubtedly, the most serious complication of surgery on the gall-bladder and biliary tract is iatrogenic bile duct injury resulting in the development of bile duct stricture. The reported incidence of this disaster is 0.25–0.5%. The more common circumstances leading to this complication include: bleeding from the right branch of the hepatic or cystic artery with blind frentic clamping of the area; excessive traction on the gallbladder and cystic duct with stenting of the common bile duct which is then inadvertently clamped; failure of appreciation of the variable anatomy of the cystic duct artery, inadequate display of the relevant anatomy; clamping of structures such as the cystic artery and duct, in preference to ligation in continuity before division. Other possible factors include devascularization of the CBD which probably accounts for the strictures encountered after CBD exploration and insertion of T-tube and leakage of bile which induces fibrosis. Whatever the exact cause, these patient if they survive, are exposed to a life time morbidity with recurrent cholangitis and jaundice. They all require major reconstructive surgery entailing transfer to centres with the necessary experience and expertise to deal with these difficult biliary problems. The outcome of these reconstructive surgical procedures depends on a number of factors, including the pathological anatomy of the stricture, the number of preceeding operations, the degree of secondary biliary cirrhosis and the presence of portal hypertension. The overall reported operative mortality from specialised centres for reconstructive surgery for bile duct strictures has been low (2–5%) and an acceptable rehabilitation rather than cure is obtained in 60–80% of cases.

Prevention

There is little doubt that the existing morbidity following biliary tract surgery can be drastically reduced if a cooperative effort is made in ensuring *safe* biliary surgery. It should be accompanied by an ongoing properly organized audit such that problems can be identified as they arise, or soon thereafter, and adequately and promptly remedied. In particular one should stress the following measures which are well recongnized but inadequately implemented.

(i) Surgical training. Aside from ensuring that our surgical trainees master the craft of surgery, we should ensure that they are taught the art of surgical exposure and that they are cognizant of the vagaries of the biliary tract anatomy. This entails a detailed knowlegde of the various congenital anomalies of the extrahepatic biliary tract and its arterial supply as well as familiarization with the corresponding cholangiographic appearances. In this respect the services of our radiological colleagues should be enlisted in the training of our surgical postgraduates.

(ii) The concept of a quick and easy cholecystec-

tomy should be taboo in surgical practice. Any biliary operation is a delicate procedure to be approached with respect, with a background of experience, the necessary intra-operative investigations and with the realization that however easy it may appear, this is an operation which hastily done could jeopardise the life of the patient or impose chronic invalidism.

(iii) Operative cholangiography should be routine without any exception. Despite the extensively reported merits of properly conducted routine operative cholangiography, this intra-operative investigation is only conducted in 30–40% of all biliary cases world wide.

(iv) The CBD should only be explored whenever necessary. Reliance only on clinical features and operative findings without cholangiography will result in overlooked stones in 5 to 10% of cases.

(v) A completion check following CBD exploration is mandatory. Most commonly this is carried out by means of a T-tube cholangiogram. Cholangioscopy is probably a more reliable alternative, although the best results are accrued from combined use of these two procedures.

Metal probing with dilators, particularly of the lower end of the CBD should be banned. The lower end of the CBD curves to the right as it transverses the head of the pancreas to enter the duodenal wall. Ill advised probing with metal rods of the Vaterian segment of the CBD during biliary tract surgery, often results in the creation of false passages with the development of fibrosis and stricture or a terminal choledocho-duodenal fistula. The sphincter region can nowadays be inspected with the choledochoscope and if probing of this region is still considered necessary it should be performed by the use of a biliary balloon catheter preferably under vision.

(vii) Finally there is nothing more counter-productive than the improper use of a recognised intra-operative investigation. Thus we should ensure familiarity with the appropriate techniques to maximize the positive yield from these investigations

The following chapters of this book deal with the principles and practicalities of investigations undertaken during the course of biliary tract surgery which allow appropriate intra-operative results in terms of patient care. The decision whether to explore the CBD or not should not be taken lightly. If the CBD requires exploration, this should be performed expeditiously and atraumatically ensuring with completion cholangiography and chol-edochoscopy against missed pathology and residual ductal calculi. Finally no amount of investigative technology absolves the surgeon from common sense and careful surgery.

CHAPTER 3

SURGICAL APPROACH AND PRINCIPLES

1. Introduction

Good surgical practice entails *careful selection* of patients for surgery whereby the predicted benefits of a surgical procedure are contrasted with the expected morbidity/mortality commensurate with age and general condition of the patient, *adequate preparation* of the patient for surgery, the use of *appropriate prophylactic measures* in patients at risk from specific complications, *safe and expeditious* surgery which entails *good exposure,* careful patient positioning and lighting, the use of intra-operative investigations when indicated *and expert postoperative care* tempered by compassion and facilitated by adequate *relief of postoperative pain.* The strict adherence to these principles is nowhere more essential than in biliary surgery. As elsewhere in surgical practice, a substancial cohort of serious complications following surgery on the biliary tract is largely preventable and the best results emanate from those centres where an obsessional attitude is adopted to prevent the preventable.

2. Prophylactic measures

The general complications which may arise in some patients during or after biliary surgery are shown in Table 3.1. By and large these occur in patients who are jaundiced and in the elderly. Thus specific prophylactic measures are unnecessary in the fit young patient undergoing elective cholecystectomy.

2.1. Infectious complications

Considerable emphasis has been made on wound infections which are often used as the end point in clinical trails concerned with evaluation of prophylactic antibiotics. Often these infections are minor and do not unduly retard convalescence.

Nevertheless strict adherence to the antiseptic ritual, gentle handling of the tissues with avoidance of tissue trauma and careful haemostasis are essential to minimize the incidence which occurs in 5 to 15% of reported series (1–3).

The clinically significant and potentially fatal complication is cholangitis which is often accompanied by septicaemia. Other infectious complications include postoperative bronchopneumonia and intra-abdominal sepsis. Postoperative chest infections arise on a background of patchy atelectasis consequent on impaired ventilation due in large measure to postoperative pain which restricts both diaphragmatic and chest wall movements.

Bacteriological studies of bile samples taken during operations have shown that positive cultures

Table 1. Complications after biliary surgery.

1.	BLEEDING	– Generalized oozing: associated with clotting factor · deficiencies and/or thrombocytopoenia
		– Arterial: cystic artery stump (slipped ligature) damaged right hepatic artery
2.	SEPSIS	– Intra-abdominal abscess formation
		– Cholangitis
		– Septicaemia
		– Bronchopneumonia
		– Wound infection
3.	BILE LEAKAGE	– Missed cut accessory duct
		– Imperfect closure of choledochotomy
		– Bile duct injury
		– Outcome: Localised collection, biliary peritonitis, external fistula
4.	MISSED PATHOLOGY	– ductal calculi high bile duct tumours
5.	IATROGENIC BILE DUCT INJURIES	– Recognised at operation Unrecognised
6.	CARDIO-VASCULAR COMPLICATIONS	– particularly in the elderly
7.	RENAL FAILURE	– in the jaundiced patient

are obtained in 45–50% of patients with acute cholecystitis, 20% of patients with chronic cholecystitis, and 75–90% of patients with jaundice caused by CBD calculi and in 30% of jaundiced patients overall. In the vast majority of patients, the organisms responsible are Gram negative aerobes (E. coli, Enterococci, Klebsiella, Pseudomonas) and anaerobic infections are rare but nevertheless do occur, are usually Clostridial and carry a high mortality (Fig. 3.1). The use of peroperative Gram staining of bile to identify those patients which require antibiotic cover (4) is of little or no value in identifying the high risk group as there is little correlation between Gram staining of bile and positive bile cultures or the incidence of postoperative infections (5). Which patients undergoing biliary tract surgery should receive antibiotic cover? There is now general agreement that prophylactic antibiotic treatment should be reserved for the high risk groups (Table 2).

Three antibiotic regimes are currently in use: Ampicillin, Ampicillin with an Aminoglycoside, or a 2nd and 3rd generation cephalosporin which is now the one most widely used. Whatever the choice, the antibiotic must be administrated at the time of induction of anaesthesia in a dose sufficient to ensure an adequate blood bacterial level during the operation. There is good evidence from prospective clinical trails that no benefit is accrued by prolonging the antibiotic therapy beyond the first two postoperative days. It is our practice to add metranidazole to the cephalosporin in patients undergoing surgery for acute cholecystitis and jaundice due to calculous obstruction of the common bile duct.

2.2. Haemorrhagic complications

A tendency to bleeding is encountered only in jaundiced patients and in patients with liver disease. In cholestatic jaundice the synthesis of the vitamin K dependent factors (II, VII, IX, and X) is impaired from malabsorption of this vitamin. In the absence of liver disease, the resultant multifactorial defect with its associated prolongation of the prothrombin time is readily reversed within 24 to 36 h by intramuscular vitamin K analogue. Failure of the prothrombin time to revert to control value indicates significant liver disease with failure of protein synthesis and a poor prognosis.

Table 2. Indications for prophylactic antibiotic therapy in biliary tract surgery

1. All jaundiced patients
2. Patients undergoing emergency operations
3. Patients over 60 years of age
4. All patients undergoing secondary biliary surgery
5. Patients with ductal calculi

In patients with secondary biliary cirrhosis the haemostatic defects are mixed and involve clotting factors, abnormal circulating anticoagulants and impaired platelet function. In the presence of portal hypertension with hypersplenism, thrombocytopenia complicates the situation further. However, haemorrhagic complications attributable to platelet deficiency are uncommon if the platelet count exceeds 50 to 60 000 per mm^3. In addition to impaired synthesis of clotting factors, there is an excess accumulation of plasminogen activators due to impaired hepatic clearance. This accounts for the frequently encountered fibrinolytic state which is compounded by the presence of an abnormal plasminogen activator produced by the diseased liver. The fibrinogen degradation products (FDP) produced by the fibrinolysis act as potent anticoagulants and also impair platelet function. Management of these patients entails the use of synthetic vitamin K, fresh frozen plasma and clotting factors concentrates. Platelet transfusions are of limited value and are only effective initially due to the development of platelet antibodies. They are therefore indicated in patients with a platelet count below 50 000 mm^3 when bleeding continues despite correction of clotting factors. Epsilon Aminocaproic Acid (EACA) is used by some to reverse the fibrinolytic state. However, its benefit is doubtful and potentially hazardous from thrombotic complications. EACA therapy should therefore be accompanied by heparin administration if the fibrinolysis is not accompanied by intravascular coagulation.

2.3. Renal failure

In biliary tract surgery renal dysfunction is encountered in patients who are jaundiced or in the presence of systemic sepsis. The pathophysiology of postoperative acute renal failure in the jaundiced patient remains unclear and it seems likely that it is multifactorial in origin. Prophylaxis consists of adequate pre-operative hydration and the induction of diuresis immediately prior to surgery with an osmotic (mannitol) or loop diuretic (frusemide). All these patients should be catheterized before surgery. A recent clinical trial has shown that pre-operative oral administration of bile salts effectively reduces the morbidity and incidence of renal failure in jaundiced patients (6).

3. Pre-operative biliary decompression in the jaundiced patient

The commonly used method of pre-operative decompression is by the percutaneous transhepatic route (Fig. 3.2) although the trans-cystic approach is used in some centres. The latter involves the insertion of a self retaining catheter into the gallbladder through the edge of the right lobe of the liver under laparoscopic guidance (Fig. 3.3). Despite its theoretical advantages and the results of early retrospective reports (7–9), there is no evidence from prospective randomized trails that this procedure reduces overall morbidity and mortality (10). Indeed there is some evidence that pre-operative decompression enhances the risk of sepsis unless a closed system of drainage is used (11). There is therefore no indication for its routine use in jaundiced patients. It seems likely, however, that the procedure may benefit patients with compromised liver function and poor nutritional state. If pre-operative external biliary decompression is used the following criteria must be followed.

(i) The decompression should be for a minimum period of 10 to 14 days.

(ii) The patients should be covered with appropriate antibiotics.

(iii) Stent dislodgement should be checked for on a daily basis.

(iv) The bile should be returned to the GI tract of the patient by means of a fine nasogastric feeding tube (Dobhof).

Internal biliary drainage methods are being increasingly used. These include insertion of an endoprosthesis by either the percutaneous transhepatic or endoscopic route. Endoscopic papillotomy is usually practised for retrieval of stones in the postoperative period but in some centres it is being performed as a pre-operative measure to relieve jaundice in patients with peri-ampullary lesions.

4. Operative principles

4.1. Surgical access.

This aspect of operative management is crucial to safe biliary surgery. Unfortunately it is not adequately taught and its importance overlooked. Its components are

(i) correct positioning of the patient on the operating table.

(ii) appropriate incision,

(iii) good illumination

(iv) efficient packing of surrounding viscera

(v) adequate exposure of relavant anatomy.

4.2. Patient positioning

The subhepatic region is relatively inaccessible particularly in obese individuals and in patients with a narrow subcostal angle. Accessibility is increased considerably if the table is broken at the level of the costal margin (approximately 30 to 40°) and at the level of the knees (circa 20°) – Figure 3.4.

4.3. Appropriate incision

Several incisions are practised. These include Kocher's (subcostal), transverse, right paramedian, midline and Mayo Robson (Fig. 3.5). Aside from individual preference, the ideal approch is dictated by the build of the patient. Thus a subcostal incision affords a rather limited access in patients with a narrow costal margin. In general a transverse incision gives good access, heals well and is the preferred approach of the author. The incision starts 2.5 cm from the mid line and courses laterally 1 cm below the costal margin well into the flank. In patients with a wide subcostal angle, it gives good access to the gallbladder and CBD and can be readily extended if necessary.

Vertical incisions are necessary in patients with a narrow subcostal angle. There is little to recommend the midline approach for biliary surgery other than speed. The incision is a weak one and access is limited particularly in obese patients.

The most widely used incision for routine cholecystectomy is the Kocher's subcostal incision. It starts just below the tip of the xiphoid process and proceeds downwards and laterally for 10 to 15 cm, 3.0 cm below and parallel to the costal margin. The 8th and 9th dorsal nerves are encountered at the lateral border of the rectus abdominis. The 8th nerve is invariably divided by this incision but the larger 9th nerve should be dissected and preserved. Subcostal causalgia is common nevertheless and carries a high nuisance value, particularly when associated with a patch of hypo/or hyperaesthesia below the costal margin. The Mayo Robson's incision consists of a vertical incision made over the centre of the upper half of the right rectus. After the anterior sheath is incised, the muscle is either retracted laterally or split in the direction of its fibres. In obese subjects and where access if limited, the upper end of the incision is prolonged inwards parallel to the costal margin, and the lower end outwards across the rectus muscle.

4.4. Illumination of the operating field

Progress in illumination technology has improved considerably over the past two decades such that in the majority of operations overhead lighting suffices. In particular the use of multiple light heads has greatly reduced the problems of shadowed areas. However, when operating on patients with narrow costal angle or when the supracolic anatomy is deeply set because of an hyperstenic build or obesity, the overhead light system often proves inadequate particularly for difficult biliary surgery. In these situations we have found the new Surgilight particularly useful. (12) The system uses a miniature xenon globe light source which produces a high intensity output with good colour temperature (5–6000 K) akin to sunlight and gives good illumination of the supra-colic compartment. The light unit itself consists of a flexible fiberoptic light cable with a reflector, interchangeable light probes and an operating table clamp with a T-bar. All the equipment can be gas sterilised, packed and stored on a mobile cart for use in the operating theatre when required. The flexible fiberoptic bundle consists of the gooseneck, the reinforced segment and the flexible part. After fixation to the operating table by means of a clamp and T-bar, the flexible gooseneck can be adjusted to the desired radius and will maintain position. The reflector and light probe is fitted and lies approximately one foot from the operating field (Figures 3.6, 3.7).

4.5. Packing

The art of packing off adjacent viscera is an attribute which facilitates display of the relevant anatomy. Opinions vary as to whether the packs should be dry or moist. What matters however is careful placement and technique of packing. In routine biliary surgery three packs are necessary. One pack is inserted to cover the left aspect of the cavity and prevent prolapse of stomach and omentum into the operating field (Fig. 3.8). The second pack is used to displace the mobilized hepatic flexure and mesocolon downwards (Fig. 3.9). The third pack covers the inferior surface of the right lobe of the liver medial to the gallbladder (Fig. 3.10). Each pack is held at one angle by a dissecting forcep until the desired depth is reached, then carefully moulded over the relevant viscera with the flat of the palm and held in place with a curved retractor positioned carefully to avoid accidental trauma.

4.6. Exposure of relevant anatomy

An adequate display of the relevant anatomy is mandatory for both primary and secondary biliary interventions. The gallbladder, liver, entire extra-hepatic biliary tract, duodenum and head of pancreas must be displayed.

(1) Display for cholecystectomy. The gallbladder may be removed by starting the dissection from the cystic duct end (retrograde) or from the fundus (anterograde). The latter approach is probably safer and should be used in difficult cases. The display varies accordingly. Preference for the anterograde approach in routine practice stems from the fact that blood loss is less than with the retrograde procedure.

Irrespective of which approach is used, a distended gallbladder is best emptied to facilitate the procedure. After the insertion of a purse string suture in the fundal region and subsequent application of a non-crushing clamp cephalad to the suture, a suction trocar cannula (Mayo Ochsner) is inserted into the gallbladder and the contents aspirated (Fig. 3.11). A specimen of the gallbladder bile/contents is sent for culture.

In anterograde cholecystectomy, the key area is the triangle of Calot. A vertical incision is made in the overlying peritoneum and by careful and gentle dissection the anatomy is displayed (Fig. 3.12). The upper bile duct is first identified, followed by the termination of the cystic duct. The cystic artery usually lies postero-superior to the duct arising from the right hepatic artery but there is considerable variation in the anatomy (see Chapter 4) and the artery should not be ligated until the following is established:

(i) The artery is seen to terminate in the gallbladder

(ii) It does not form a loop curving up to the liver since this course is often that of an aberrant right hepatic artery with the cystic branch originating from the apex of the loop.

It is good practice whenever possible to ligate (or clip) and divide the cystic artery before the cystic duct. The main reason for this policy is to prevent traction rupture of the cystic artery during ligation of the cystic duct, the torn artery retracting into the porta hepatis. In practice, however, ligation and division of the cystic duct is often performed first as this facilitates access to the artery and provided ligatures are inserted around the duct without the application of clamps, the eventuality described above becomes extremely remote (Fig. 3.13).

(2) Additional exposure for exploration of CBD. It is essential in all these cases that a complete mobilization of the duodenum is carried out. Without this mobilization a reliable exploration of the extrahepatic biliary tract particularly the lower end of the bile duct and operative cholangioscopy is not possible (Chapter 5). The technique of duodenal mobilization is described in Chapter (7).

(3) Exposure for secondary biliary intervention. Whether performed for missed/recurrent stones or iatrogenic stricture, this intervention requires experience and is often technically difficult. As expected secondary procedures carry a higher morbidity and mortality which are however dependent on the underlying pathology, the number of previous surgical interventions, general condition and age of the patient.

Inevitably dense adhesions are found in the supracolic compartment particularly in the right hypochondrium involving the liver, diaphragm, duodenum, hepatic flexure, omentum and anterior abdominal wall. The division of these adhesions must proceed in a systematic manner as follows:

(i) Division of anterior adhesions involving liver and adjacent viscera to the anterior abdominal wall starting medially and proceeding in a lateral direction.

(ii) Separation of right lobe of the liver from diaphragm, omentum, hepatic flexure followed by division of ligamentum teres.

(iii) Mobilization of the hepatic flexure and adjacent colon which are then reflected downwards and medially.

(iv) Mobilization of the duodenal bulb which is often found adherent to the porta hepatis. This is followed by complete mobilization of second and third parts of the duodenum together with the pancreatic head.

(v) Identification of the lower end of the common bile duct after pancreatico-duodenal mobilization. The duct is then followed proximally.

(vi) In the case of bile duct strictures, dissection of the fibrous plaque leading to the porta hepatis is required to identify a mucosa lined proximal bile duct. This dissection is hazardous and requires considerable experience and familiarity with the pathological anatomy.

5. Drainage of the supracolic compartment after biliary operations

This seemingly controversial issue is best discussed in relation to the nature of the biliary operation performed.

(1) After Cholecystectomy. Whereas few would argue against the use of drainage in patients with excessive oozing of blood or bile spillage during surgery, acute suppurative, gangrenous or perforated cholecystitis, in the debilitated or immunosuppressed, controversy exists as to the need of drainage after an uneventful elective cholecstectomy. It would seem that the argument against drainage has been strengthened by the results of two prospective clinical trails (13, 14). Both studies failed to show any material benefit from drainage. However these trials have one severe limitation which precludes safe conclusions. This relates to number of patients entered into the study, 50 in each group. The incidence of unexpected bile leakage after elective cholecystectomy without bile duct exploration averages 0.5%. It is therefore obvious that with the numbers involved, it is mathematically impossible to detect a difference and indeed in both studies not a single case of bile leak was observed in the drainage and non-drainage groups. It seems likely that for the vast majority of these patients, it

matters little if drains are inserted or not but one in every 200 patients will develop a postoperative bile leak with disastrous consequences if the surgeon omitted to insert a subhepatic drain. Common sense dicates that such a rare eventuality is one too many. In the author's opinion the avoidance of drainage offers no particular benefit to patients after cholecystectomy and can expose the occasional patient to an otherwise avoidable complication.

(2) After CBD exploration and secondary biliary intervention. There is no controversy regarding the need for drainage in these cases. Opinion differs as to whether the subhepatic pouch alone or together with the right subdiaphragmatic region should be drained. Some favour sump suction drains, other Penrose, Redivac or tube drains. The author's preference is for silicone tube drains leading to a closed system (Fig. 3.14) with drainage of the subhepatic pouch only after a straightforward bile duct exploration and drainage of both the subdiaphragmatic space and subhepatic pouch after more major biliary surgery.

References

1. Cox JF, Helfrich LR, Pass HI, Osterhaut S, Shingelton WW: The relationship between biliary tract infections and postoperative complications. Surg Gynec Obstet 146: 233–236, 1978.

2. Pyrtek LJ, Bartus SA: An evaluation of antibiotics in biliary tract surgery. Surg Gynec Obstet 127: 101–105, 1967.

3. Fyfe AHB, Mohammed R, Dougall AJ: The infective complications of elective cholecystectomy. Operative biliary infection related to post-operative complications. J Roy Coll Surg Ed 28: 90–95, 1983.

4. McLeish AR, Keighley MR, Bishop HM et al.: Selecting patients requiring antibiotics in biliary surgery by immediate Gram stain of bile at Operation. Surgery 81: 473–477, 1977.

5. Gallagher P, Ostick G, Jones D. Schofield PF, Tweedle DE: Intra operative bile microscopy. Is it useful? Brit J Surg 69: 473–474, 1982.

6. Evans HJR, Torrealba V, Hudd C, Knight M: The effect of pre-operative bile salt administration on postoperative renal function in patients with obstructive jaundice. Br J Surg 69:706–708.

7. Nakayama T, Ikeda A, Okuda R: Percutaneous transhepatic drainage of the biliary tract. Gastroenterology 74:544–599, 1978.

8. Ishikawa Y, Oishi L, Miyai M et al.: Percutaneous transhepatic drainage: experience in 100 cases. J. Clin Gastroenterol 2:305–314, 1980.

9. Mori K, Misumi A, Sugiyama M, et al.: Percutaneous transhepatic bile drainage. Ann Surg 185:111–115, 1977.

10. Hatfield ARW, Tobias R, Terblance J, et al.: Preoperative external biliary drainage in obstructive jaundice. Lancet ii:896–899, 1982.

11. McPherson GHD, Benjamin IS, Habib NGA, Bowley NB, Blumgart LH: Percutaneous transhepatic drainage in obstructive jaundice: advantages and problems. Br J Surg 69:261–264, 1982.

12. Berci G, Cuschieri A: A new auxiliary universal surgi-light. Br J Surg 71: 160, 1984.

13. Gordon AB, Bates T, Fiddian V: A controlled trial of drainage after cholecystectomy. Br J Surg 63:278–282, 1976.

14. Trowbridge PE: A randomized study of cholecysteetomy with and without drainage. Surg Gynec Obstet 155:171–176, 1982.

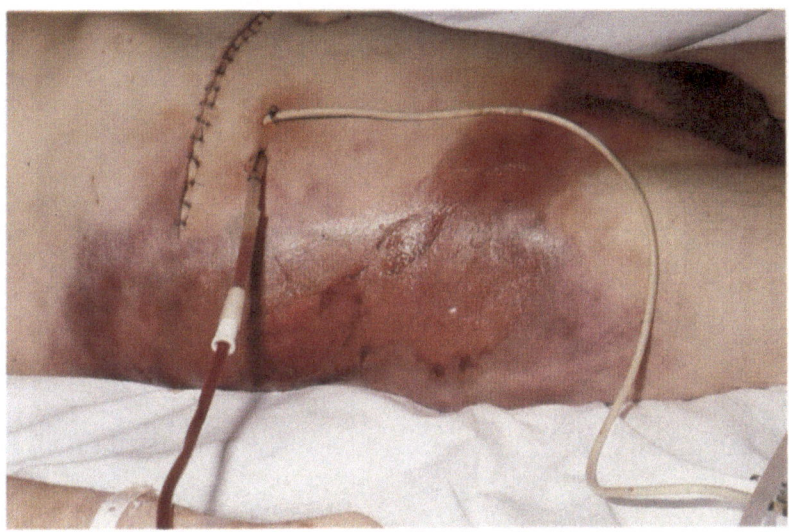

Fig. 3.1. Gas gangrene developing after cholecystectomy and exploration of the CBD in 62 years old male. The infection became clinically apparent with obvious gangrene and crepitus on the third post-operative day and proved fatal.

Cl. welchii organisms were grown from the exudate.

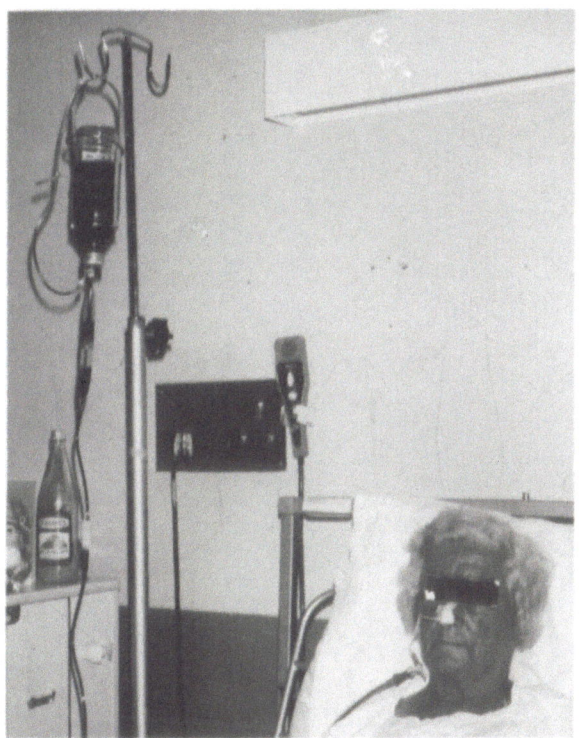

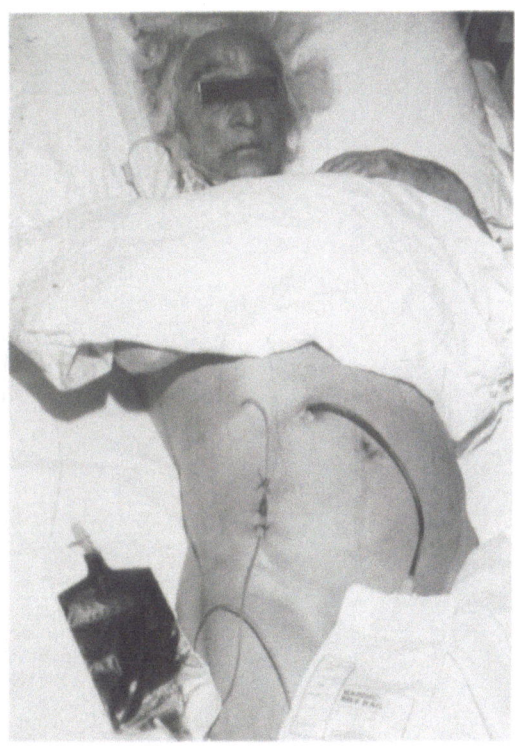

Fig. 3.2. External (percutaneous) transhepatic decompression in a 70 year old female with total bile duct obstruction caused by a hilar carcinoma (Klatskin tumour). The importance of a closed system of drainage to prevent infection is now well established. The collected bile is infused into the GI tract via a fine feeding (Dobhof) tube. The decompression was maintained for 2 weeks with considerable improvement in the general condition of the patient and virtual subsidance of the jaundiced state. The patient then underwent an uneventful excision of the hilar tumour and is alive and well 2 years later.

Fig. 3.3. Laparoscopic decompression an an elderly female who presented with severe jaundice, cholangitis and septicaemia. The laparoscopic cholangiogram showed obstruction caused by a single solitary calculus. After 10 days of decompression and antibiotic therapy (cephuroxime and metranidazole), the patient underwent successful cholecystectomy, exploration of CBD and removal of impacted calculus under visual control by the cholangioscope.

14

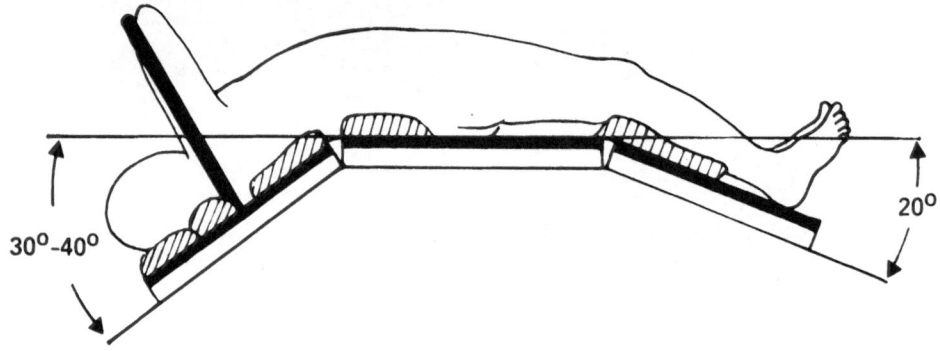

Fig. 3.4. Patient positioning for biliary surgery. With the patient in a supine position, the table is broken at the level of a costal margin, this enhances access particularly in patients with a narrow subcostal angle. The table is also broken at the level of the knee joints to prevent slipping.

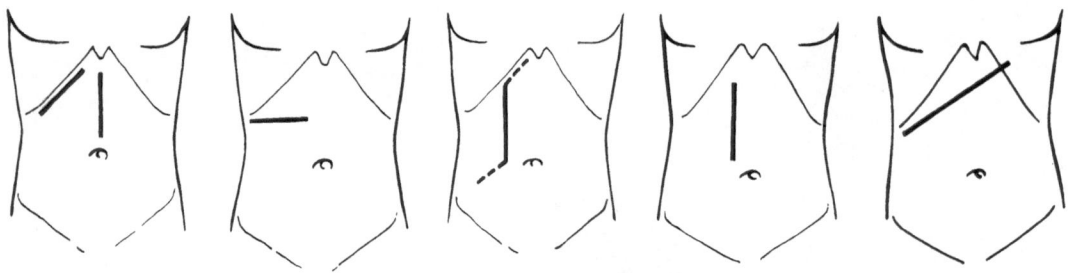

Fig. 3.5. Incisions used for biliary surgery. A thoraco-abdominal approach is rarely necessary.

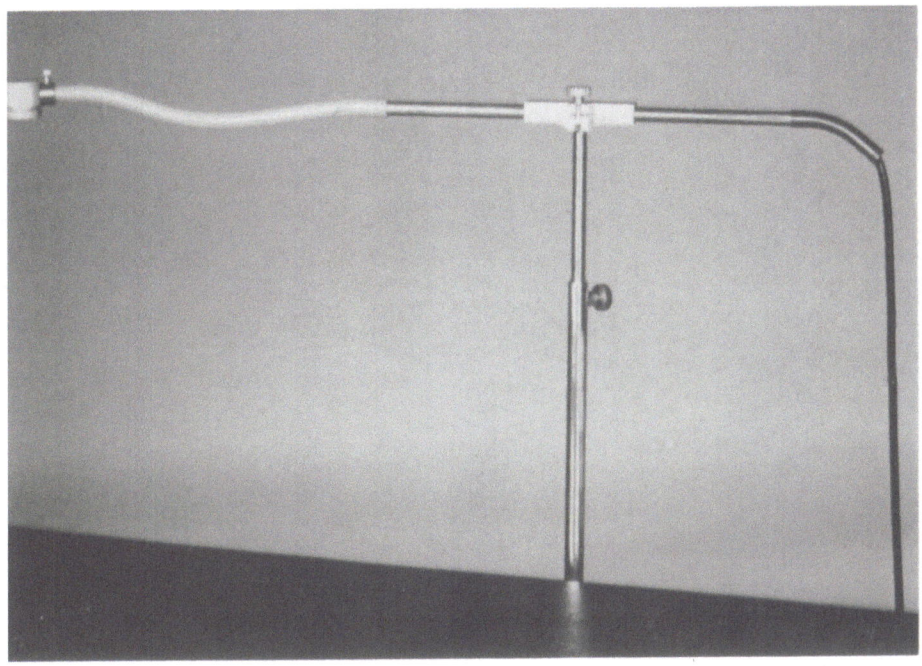

Fig. 3.6. Assembled surgilight fitted with reflector.

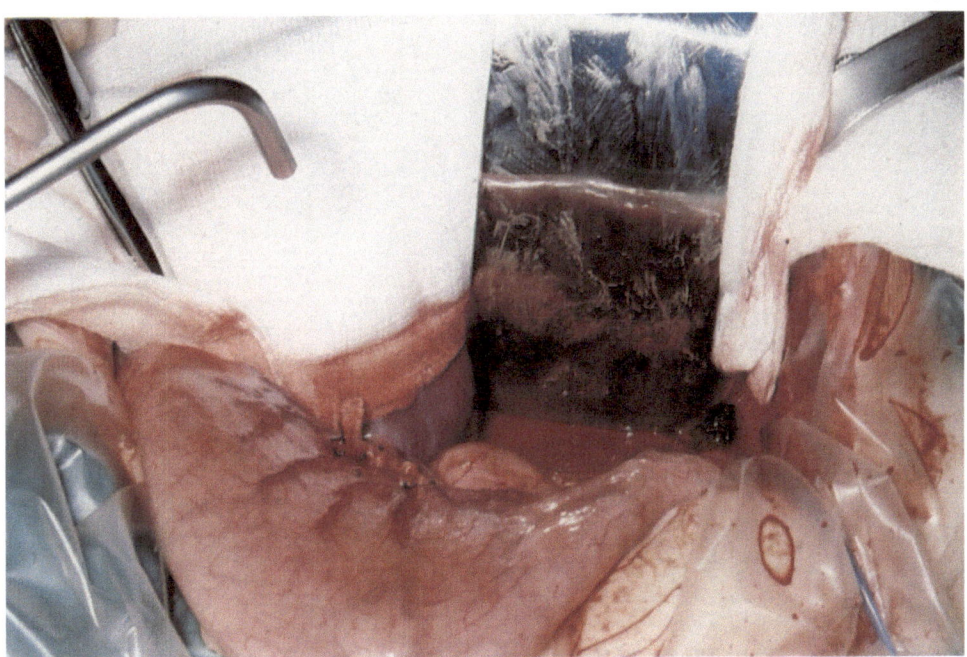

Fig. 3.7. Extra illumination of the operating field by surgilight fitted with the angled light probe.

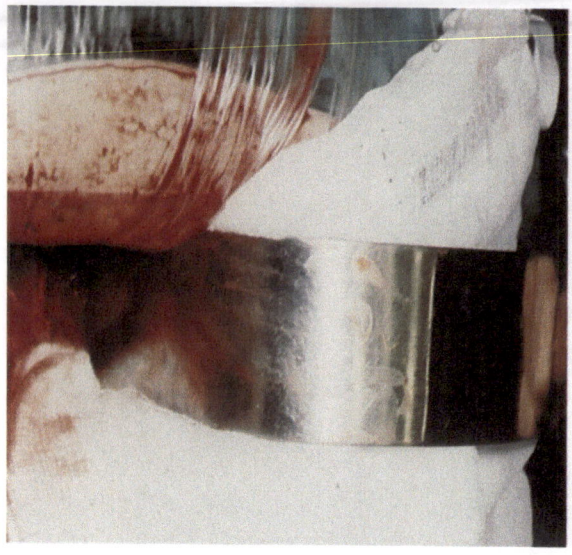
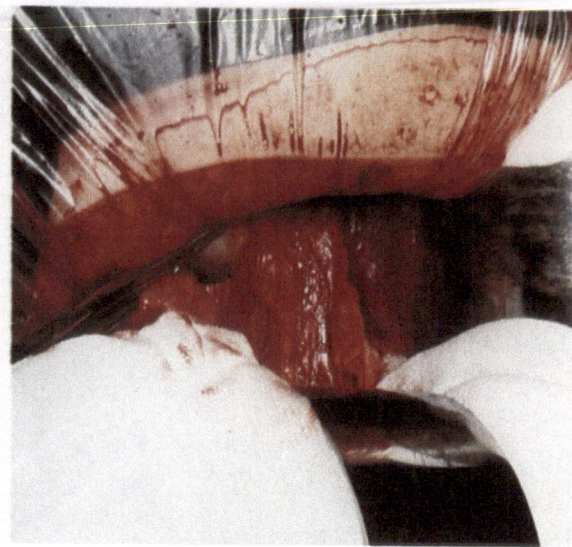

Fig. 3.8. Packing for biliary surgery. Pack inserted to cover left aspect of supracolic compartment preventing prolapse of stomach and omentum into the operating field.

Fig. 3.9. Packing for biliary surgery. Second pack is used to displace the mobilized hepatic flexure and mesocolon downwards.

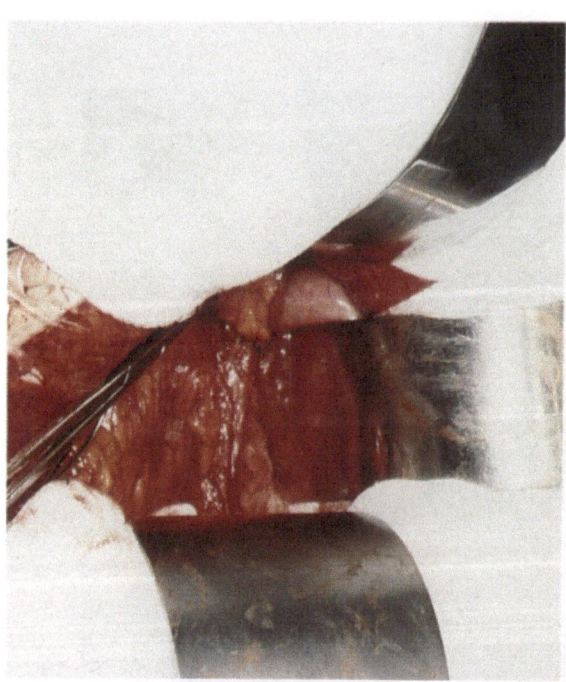
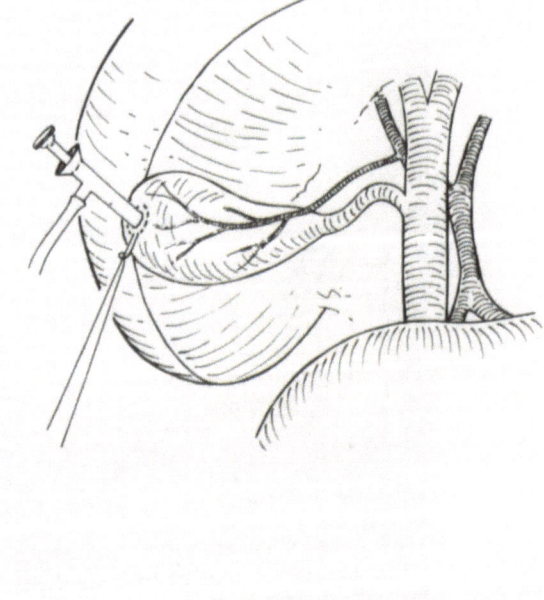

Fig. 3.10. Packing for biliary surgery. The third pack is inserted to cover the inferior surface of the right lobe of the liver to protect it from retractor trauma.

Fig. 3.11. Technique of gallbladder aspiration which is used where a tense distended gallbladder is found at laparotomy.

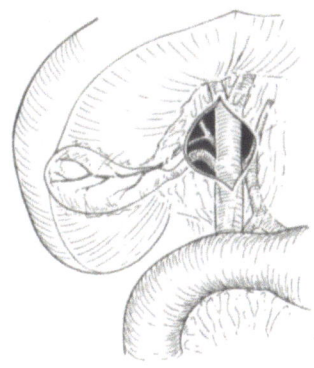

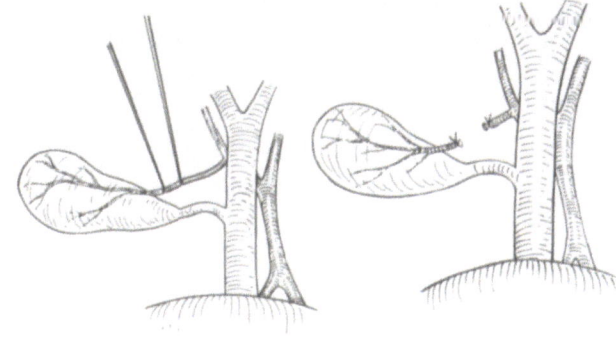

Fig. 3.12. Anatomy of the triangle of Calot. An appreciation of the anatomy of this key area and the possible congenital aberrations is crucial for safe biliary surgery.

Fig. 3.13a. Technique of ligation of the cystic artery without the application of haemostatic clamps. Alternatively the artery may be Liga clipped and then divided.

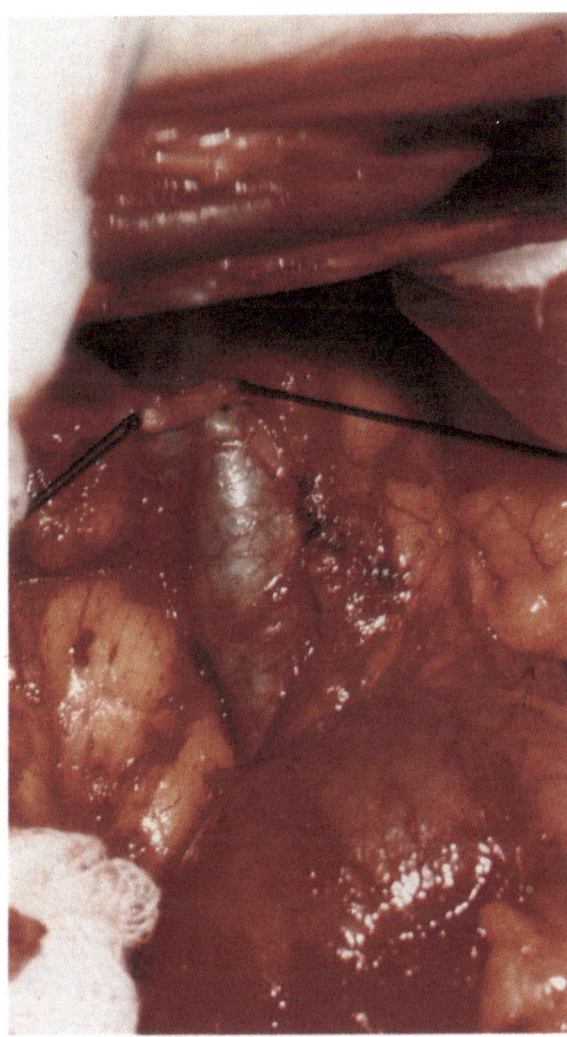

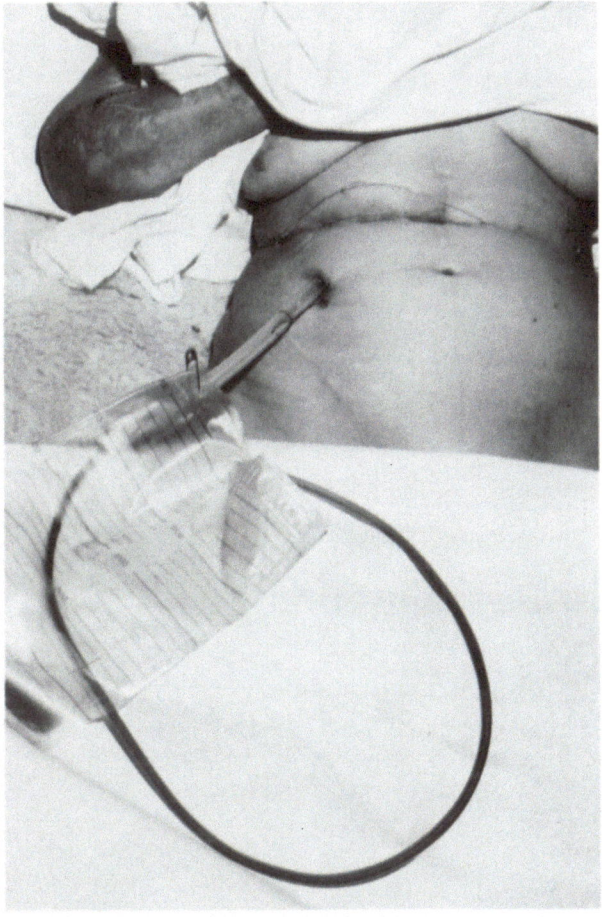

Fig. 3.13b. The cystic artery is shown ligated at each end prior to division. The cystic duct is seen just below the artery. Often the duct is ligated before the artery using a similar technique.

Fig. 3.14. Silicone tube closed drainage system for use in operations on the biliary tract. A transverse incision favoured by the author for routine cholecystectomy ± exploration of the CBD has been done.

CHAPTER 4

OPERATIVE CHOLANGIOGRAM

1. Introduction

Intraoperative cholangiography was introduced by Mirrizi a half century ago (1, 2). Although this important intraoperative modality has been available for decades, there has been little effort made to improve the technique and to encourage its greater use (3, 4, 5). Surgeons continue to be sceptical about routine cholangiography because they claim that it is too time consuming, its technical failure rate is unacceptably high, as is its false-positive or false-negative rate, and furthermore, it is not cost effective (6, 7, 8).

Operative cholangiography has been an 'orphan', trying to find a home between two families: surgeons and radiologists. When it falls short of expectations, surgeons point to the radiologist, blaming equipment failure, poor exposure techniques, developing time delay and interpretative errors and therefore feel frustrated by the lack of understanding and control of radiological factors.

Radiologists consider the examination as substandard because they lack direct control, blaming the surgeons for not understanding the basic techniques, such as the necessity of scout films, the importance of patient positioning, careful injection of contrast material, and the removal of foreign bodies (clamps, retractors, NG tubes, swabs, etc.) from the field.

If progress is to be achieved, a *cooperative effort must be made* by both disciplines to the ultimate benefit of the patient.

In many hospitals, geographical separation of the operating rooms and X-ray department means that the radiographer or the radiologist must travel between the two locations to evaluate films and communicate with personnel. If direct discussion about the findings is necessary, the radiologist must change before entering the operating room proper,

which further prolongs the procedure. Installation of an inexpensive audio-intercommunication system between the two departments could help to alleviate this delay. Surgeons are not trained in the radiological interpretation and although many have developed a skill for reading their own cholangiograms, the difficult or troublesome case requires the trained eye of the radiologist to assist in intraoperative decision making (9). For this reason operative cholangiography should be regarded as a *procedure requiring the presence or availability of the radiologist.*

Outdated protable X-ray machines are frequently relegated to surgery and thereby a double standard of film quality is established between the operating rooms and radiology department. X-ray film quality means maximum information available and is in proportion to the diagnostic accuracy. The degree of equipment sophistication should be related to the size of the hospital as well as the volume and type of surgery requiring radiographic assistance. The radiologist should help in obtaining the best radiologic equipment available in order to optimize patient care. The initial capital outlay, maintenance, and operating costs for permanently installed equipment are justified in hospitals where the yearly surgical volume of biliary cases (150–200) and orthopedic operations (500–1 000) is high and where other procedures, such as cardiac pacemaker and parenteral alimentation catheter placements, are frequent. The cost of more expensive equipment (one fixed installation is equal to approximately three or four portable units) must also be weighted against *the expense incurred by the individual who suffers a complication* such as a retained stone *requiring prolonged hospitalization or repeated procedures* (see Chapter 8 Postoperative Removal of Retained Stones Through the T-tube Tract) or iatrogenic injuries (Fig. 4.1) that

20

might have been avoided if optimal operative radiology would have been available. Another economic factor to consider is the *decrease in operating time* (utilization of operating rooms) that is the result of improved operating radiology thus permitting a more rapid turnover of operating room cases.

2. Common bile duct explorations

In 15 to 20% of all biliary operations the common bile duct is explored. The indications for common bile duct (CBD) exploration include: history of jaundice, pancreatitis, demonstration of multiple stones within the gallbladder with a dilated cystic duct, dilated CBD, and palpable stones within the CBD. Unfortunately, *the incidence of negative explorations is high (20 to 40%)* when these clinical criteria are the sole indications for opening the duct (10, 11).

3. Unsuspected stones

The incidence of unsuspected ductal calculi is 4 to 10% (12, 13). In our experience of 500 consecutive simple cholecystectomies, we found stones in the extra-hepatic biliary system in 25 cases (5%) without past or present history of jaundice and normal biochemical assays (14). These were only discovered by employing a serial film technique which permits observing the early filling stage (for details see below) and by employing proper cholangiography *as a routine.*

4. Cannulation techniques

A variety of cannulae and instruments have been developed for injecting the extra-hepatic biliary system during surgery. The following criteria should be fulfilled:

(a) The insertion of any cannula into the duct system should be simple and not time consuming.

(b) The actual cannulation should be performed under direct visual control.

(c) Securing the cannula, or needle, should not be difficult technically. Leakage or inadvertent dislodging has to be prevented.

In 1972 we advocated the use of a hemoclip to fix a Fr. 5 Lehman radio-opaque catheter in the cystic duct (15). It was easier than trying a knot in the great depth. Care had to be taken, however, to avoid having the metal clip compress the lumen of the catheter, which occurred occasionally.

Subsequently we found that employing a metal 'S'-shaped cannula to be preferable (Figs. 4. 2a–c) (16). Because of the offset between the hub and tip of the cannula, the latter remains clearly visible when introduced and it is not obscured by the guiding hand. Fixation is achieved by a right angled clamp, similar to the one described by Borge (17). For equivalent outer diameters the lumen of the metal cannula is larger than the plastic catheter because of the thinner wall, and therefore, the resistance to injection pressure is less. This is an important consideration when obtaining manometric measurements (see Chapter 6).

Any cannulation system to be employed should be carefully rinsed to expel all air bubbles (Fig. 4.2d). A venous extension tube joins the cannula to a stopcock with two syringes, one containing contrast material (glass syringe) and the other saline (plastic syringe). We use syringes of different materials to avoid confusion as to their contents. After carefully removing all air bubbles from the system the change over from saline to contrast is made by a stopcock, rather than by exchanging syringes and inadvertently introducing air bubbles. The practice of aspirating the cannula after its insertion into the bile duct is inadvisable as it often results in duodenal air being sucked into the CBD.

From the standpoint of radiology, attention must be given to two points:

(a) A film should be taken prior to contrast injection to document the position of the cannula.

(b) Extravasation of contrast material from the site of cannulation entry can interfere with radiographic interpretation (Fig. 4.2e). It is much easier to reposition a metal cannula that is held by a right angled clamp than to attempt to unite a knot or release a clip deep in the wound to adjust a plastic catheter.

5. Initial and/or completion cholangiograms

Optimally both initial and completion cholangiograms should be performed. If circumstances allow only one procedure, the initial cystic duct cholangiogram (or in case of a secondary exploration, the primary choledochocholangiogram) *is preferred* because of dealing with a closed system without artifacts caused by manipulation. Initial cystic duct cholangiography provides much information to the surgeon, *early in the course of the operation*. The timely display of ductal anatomy aids in subsequent dissection. Attention will be drawn to important anomalies of surgical interest (8%) and the number and location of stones will be indicated. With a well performed negative cholangiogram, unnecessary exploration of the common bile duct accompanied by an increased morbidity rate can be avoided.

The completion cholangiogram is often more difficult to interpret than the initial one. Following duct exploration, air bubbles may be incompletely evacuated (Fig. 4.3a). After prolonged manipulation or stone extraction attempts, desquamative or cholangitic debris and blood clots may produce radiolucencies, obscuring or simulating a calculus (Fig. 4.3b), thereby reducing the confidence level in film interpretation. *These are the cases where operative biliary endoscopy can solve the dilemma*. The initial or preliminary cholangiogram is therefore more reliable because it is performed in a *closed system* prior to introduction of *potential artifacts*.

6. Standard technique

6.1. Technique and equipment

The orthodox 2 to 3 film cholangiogram is usually performed with a portable X-ray machine. In many instances it is a unit that has been 'retired' from service on the floor and given to surgery. Consequently the performance of this unit may be suboptimal. The production of an adequate abdominal radiograph with the portable equipment is difficult at best, and patients with cholelithiasis are often overweight, which adds to the technical limitations. Therefore, an X-ray machine with greater capacity is recommended to achieve a satisfactory image with a shorter exposure time. An exposure with a 300 mA portable unit is sufficient for most non-obese patients.

A hospital with five or six operating theaters for general and orthopedic surgery should obtain such a machine dedicated for operating room use only. The time delays that frequently occur in calling for a portable machine to be brought in form another area prolongs the anesthesia time unnecessarily.

Various film cassette holding devices have been designed for use with the standard operating room table. Tables are now available with radiolucent tabletops and built-in cassette holders, or tunnels. In either case, access to the film cassette is difficult with sterile drapes hanging over the side of the table. The use of a grid will improve the film quality during standard cholangiography and slightly increases the required radiation dose. Its use, however, requires precise alignment of the tube and grid by the technician to avoid interfering grid lines. Unless the grid is oriented transverse to the patient, lateral tilting of the table with film cassette and grid in the tunnel will severely degrade the quality of the film.

6.2. Patient's positioning

With the patient supine, the common bile duct is often projected over the spine contributing to the difficulties in visualizing or assessing the CBD (Fig. 4.4). A 10°–15° rotation of the patient to the right is required to avoid superimposing the CBD and vertebrae. Some tables can be tilted to the side, otherwise radiolucent wedges or sponges, rolled linen, or inflatable cuffs can be placed under the patient's left flank to achieve the needed obliquity.

Because of the uncertainty in positioning, the film used for standard cholangiography is larger than necessary to display the biliary system. An 11×14 inch film, but more often a 14×17 inch format, is used to ensure that the common bile duct will appear somewhere on the film. The X-ray collimator is fulled openend to expose the entire film, losing the advantage of a narrow coning and better film quality.

6.3. Scout film

A preliminary scout film prior to commencing surgery aids the radiographer in assessing the appropriate exposure required for each patient. Not doing so leaves the technical adequacy of a film to chance.

6.4. Injected volume

It is impossible to predict the volume of the biliary system in the individual case. Small ducts may be filled with 5–10 ml of contrast material whereas dilated ducts may require 20–50 ml.

The sphincter tone can also influence the degree of filling. A relaxed sphincter results in immediate opacification of the duodenum with little or no visualization of proximal ducts. When the opposite occurs, the ducts are overfilled and the degree of opacity within the ducts may obscure small stones. Excessive injection pressure may rupture small intra-hepatic ducts. An injection schedule has been adopted for the CBD which measures up to 10 mm diameter. Exposures follow injection of 3 ml, 5 ml, and 10 ml contrast material. Surprising success folows this 'blind' injection technique, but it is undoubtedly inferior to visually controlled injection of contrast material and the important early stage is missed in the majority of cases (Fig. 4.5) (18, 19).

6.5. Contrast material

We prefer a 25% solution of Hypaque (Sodium diatrizoate). Although further diluted by the CBD bile, this concentration allows X-ray penetration suffient to visualize small calculi within the duct. A range 70–80 kV used. Others have suggested higher kilo voltage to achieve greater penetration of the contrast column (20). This may be useful when larger volumes of contrast material are employed. If automatic exposure control is available, density on the film is better controlled.

6.6. Coordination of exposure

Great care must be exercised in the cannulation and injection technique so as not to introduce air, which could be mistaken for calculi. It is essential for the anesthesiologist to produce complete apnea of the patient during exposure, an exercise which is not always completely successful but is required to avoid motion when longer exposure times are employed.

6.7. Mobile C-arm Fluoroscope

Orthopedic surgeons introduced the mobile image amplifier with television fluoroscopy for trauma surgery. During reduction of fractures the films are exposed only to identify the position of the frag-

ments and to determine what steps should be taken. There is no real need for permanent documentation in this manipulative phase. A quick look on the television screen gives the indication to continue or to terminate the procedure. The time consuming procedure of exposure, processing and waiting are excluded. The further incorporation of the static image storage system decreases further radiation exposure

It is also employed by thoracic surgeons (pacemaker insertions), localization of catheter insertions, radio-opaque foreign body removals. etc.

This equipment is built *as a mobile unit*. Its configuration is ideal for obtaining antero-posterior or oblique views by moving the aligned X-ray tube and image amplifier with the television camera on the C-circle. Because of the mobility, the weight and therefore the generator and tube have to be kept *small*. A radiograph can be made by sliding a film cassette holder in the image amplfer. This machine *cannot afford the delivery of a larger X-ray dosage in a shorter period of time*. In case of stationary objects (extremities), the exposure time is not a great problem. For the abdomen, these units are not very satisfactory because of the same problem or shortcomings which are encountered with the standard portable unit in radiography. The fluoroscopic image information is of help, but not enough to make a precise diagnosis in the display of the extrahepatic biliary system. The exposure times for a radiograph of the abdomen in an obese patient is far too long.

7. Fluoro-cholangiography

Because of the limitations of abdominal radiology using portable technique, significant further improvement in film quality and diagnostic accuracy in standard operative cholangiography *seems unlikely*. If advancement is to be made, investment in equipment of greater capacity, requiring fixed installation, should be seriously considered. Consistently reliable and adequate radiographic examinations are required for the operating room just as they are in the radiology department. By providing the surgeon with *accurate information in a timely manner* the incidence of complications (missed stones, iatrogenic injuries) can be reduced.

We have developed a fluoro-cholangiographic technique which we believe is superior to the standard method. The case load in our institution (Cedars-Sinai Medical Centre) requires the examination of 250–300 operative biliary cases per year. Since critical decisions are based on cholangiographic findings we felt that the examination ought to be of the same high quality as the postoperative T-tube examination performed in the X-ray department. This required the installation of special equipment (Figs. 4.6a–f) designed to provide both radiographic and fluoroscopic images.

A three phase generator with 800–1000 mA capicity is needed. The transformer and control panel are placed in a clean corridor between two operating rooms. The X-ray tube is permanently mounted in the operating rooms and can be swung to the side and out of the way when not in use (Fig. 4.6b). The X-ray tube and the image amplifier (IA) may be joined by the C-arm as one unit (Fig. 4.6c) or the IA can be brought into position under the operating room table and fixed in place by floor mounts while the overhead tube is swung to the pre-determined position directly above the IA (Fig. 4.6d). The positioning requires only a short period of time and is always optimally aligned. The time consuming maneuvering and alignment procedures of a portable unit are thereby eliminated.

Employing indirect radiography, 100×100 mm cut films are used in a camera providing a permanent film record. Fluoroscopy is observed on a mobile floor or ceiling mounted television monitor in the operating room, as well as simultaneously on a remote monitor in the X-ray department (Fig. 4.6e). A double foot switch (Fig. 4.6f) allows the surgeon to control both the fluoroscopy and film exposures. Two additional pieces of equipment are necessary. A surgical table with a radiolucent top which can be moved in a coordinate (x-y) fashion ensures fast and precise centralization of the objects under scrutiny (Fig. 4.6c). In addition, an automatic film processor located within the surgical suite further facilitates the rapid completion of the examination and the viewing of *dry* films within minutes. The advantages of fluoro-cholangiography over the standard technique includes the following important factors:

7.1. Easy positioning of the patient
The ability to observe the fluoroscopic image permits minor changes in the position of the patient using the floating coordinate tabletop. These adjustments can be made even during the examination. Interfering foreign bodies discovered on the television screen (retractor, sponges, NG tube, etc.) can be removed before the contrast injection is started (Figs. 4.7a–d).

7.2. Optimal beam collimation
When the technician is certain of the patient's position and is sure that the CBD is central to the beam, the shutter can be approximated to improve image quality.

7.3. Shorter exposure time
The greater capacity of the quipment results in a shorter exposure time (1/20th to 1/30th of a second) *so that blurring due to motion is avoided.* Even in the obese patient, it is unnecessary for the anesthesiologist to suspend respiration during the exposure.

7.4. Automatic exposure control
Photo-timing of exposures provides uniformity of film quality. Photo-timing is not generally available with portable equipment.

7.5. Minimal technician activity
The movements of the technician within the operating room is minimized since there is no exchange of cassettes between exposures. The film receiver is removed from the head of the table when the examination is completed. No lifting up of sterile towels or interference with the sterile area is imposed. It is important to decrease unnecessary traffic of non-surgical personnel, to avoid contamination of sterile areas.

7.6. Control of the exposure sequence
The timing of each exposure is determined by observing the degree of *ductal opacification* (filling stages) fluoroscopically. The need for repeating the examination because of overfilling or underfilling of the duct is avoided.

7.7. Serial films

The examination is not limited to two or three exposures, and in fact, the serial film technique is recommended using 6 to 12 exposures and emphasizing the need to see the early filling phase (Figs. 4.8a–h). The acquisition of multiple films taken during the course of the injection is helpful in clarifying the nature of some puzzling artifacts or abnormalities encountered on cholangiograms. *Our average is 10.4 films per patient.*

7.8. Decreased examination time

Having dispensed with the exchange of film cassettes for each exposure and the wheeling in and centering of the equipment, the total examination time *is drastically reduced.* The entire cholangiographic process, including slow injection, interrupted fluoroscopy and serial films, can be completed within 5 to 6 minutes. The need for repeated injections because of technical problems is almost completely eliminated.

7.9. Indirect radiography

The use of the film camera contributes to a relatively compact unit more suitable to an operating room environment. Objections have been raised to interpreting the image on the smaller 100 × 100 mm (4 × 4 inches) film, based on the belief that insufficient detail is obtained. This has not been so in practice.

Even minute intra-hepatic branches can be easily seen (Fig. 4.9). We have identified and documented calculi as small as 2–3 mm within a normal sized common bile duct. Image enlargement on the film can be obtained if the IA tube is constructed with the capacity of electronic magnificantion (Figs. 4.8e and h). The resolution of a 100 × 100 mm film is more than sufficient for cholangiography. In many radiology departments this film technique is employed for angiography (two to six films per second) and has proved to be sufficient in detail.

8. Anomalies of surgical importance

We emphasize the necessity of obtaining topographic information early in the course of the operation, by performing an initial cholangiogram. An important and often unexpected anatomic detail can be displayed (21).

8.1. Short cystic duct

If this duct is short or near the main duct and covered by fibrous sheets or edematous tissues, the surgeon knows that the cysticus has to be carefully ligated near the cannulation-incision (Figs. 4.10a–b).

8.2. Drainage of cystic duct in the right hepatic duct

The cystic duct may join the right hepatic duct within the liver or in the porta. More frequently the cystic duct unites with an aberrant right hepatic duct to drain together into the common bile duct (Figs. 4.11a–b). If this is unrecognized, the patient may suffer from a ligated or divided hepatic branch.

8.3. Aberrant ducts

The drainage of a right hepatic branch from either the cephalic or caudal division may join the common duct near the cystic duct entry (Fig. 4.12). If this 'extra' duct in the Calot's triangle is divided and not recognized, a postoperative biliary fistula can result . A similar situation may occur if there is a division of a duct communicating directly with the gallbladder. Only careful dissection of the gallbladder bed or possibly cholecystocholangiography would identify this anomaly.

8.4. Ductal diverticula and choledochocele

Small stones may enter a ductal diverticulum and may be difficult to remove. Endoscopy may overlook a stone within this pouch. The presence of a choledochocele is associated with an increasing incidence of common duct calculi and a sphincteroplasty should be considered (Figs. 4.13a–b).

8.5. The acute or emergency case

These are difficult patients due to circumstances, time factors, anatomy and other aspects. In these technically delicate situations with critically ill patients, a cholangiogram can provide a road map. If the icterus is associated with septicemia, a well displayed choledochogram can differentiate between jaundice due to distal mechanical obstruction or bacteremia. With a severely ill patient, it is essential to avoid extending the operation with increased morbidity and mortality (Figs. 4.14a–e).

9. General aspects

The key to successful functioning of the system is the *close collaboration between the radiologist and the surgeon*. The technician tests the equipment and takes the scout films while the anesthesiologist prepares the patient. The radiologist is then alerted that the surgery is starting. As the surgeon prepares for the cystic duct cannulation, the technician notifies the radiologist that the examination is imminent. The radiologist observes the fluoroscopy on the remote monitor in the X-ray department and gives necessary instructions over the intercom system to be sure that the cholangiogram is performed adequately. As soon as the films are processed, the radiologist reviews the developed film and writes his/her findings in the progress notes of the chart, thus avoiding a later debate or confusion as to what was said. The surgeon may remove the gallbladder leaving the cystic duct cannula in place while awaiting the films and the radiologist's report. If for some reason the examination is not satisfactory or there is uncertainty, additional exposures should be taken. The radiologist should not hesitate to ask for repeat films. In doubtful cases, with this equipment, it takes only a few minutes to have another series of film available.

10. Radiation protection

Appropriate precautions should be taken to minimize radiation exposure to all personnel as well as to the patient. During the procedure the surgeon should wear a gas sterilized lead apron. If sterilization is not possible he can double gown or double glove, but a lead apron must be worn. A venous extension tube will allow the surgeon to step back three or four feet during the injection thereby further reducing his exposure. The anesthesiologist must also wear a lead apron and should not leave the patient. The scrub nurse and surgical assistant should be behind a protective screen in one corner of the room. Non-sterile personnel should step out of the room.

Film budges are worn by all personnel in the operating room to monitor exposure. Fluoroscopic time is reported for each case and the surgeons are cautioned to keep the time to a minimum by maintaining a 'light foot' (i.e. intermittent short fluoroscopic exposures). These protective measures require little effort and are very worthwhile. With the increasing number of diagnostic procedures requiring radiographic assistance and exposure to personnel working within the hospital, it is important to remember that radiation doses are cumulative (22).

11. The cystic duct

Our study of the cystic duct has revealed a significant deviation from the standard concept of its course in relationship to the common duct (Fig. 4.15). In our series, we have found that the cystic duct entered the right lateral side of the common duct in *only 17% of the patients*. In 41% the duct entered the anterior or posterior aspects of the common duct. Of particular interest was that in 35% of the patients the cystic duct passed around the choledochus posteriorly to enter the medial aspect of the common bile duct. These are referred to as spiral cystic ducts (Figs. 4.16a–b). A long parallel drainage was seen only in 7% of the patients. Thus in a *high percentage of cases* (83%) the cystic duct stump lateral to the common bile duct constitutes only a fraction of its total length. The incidence of a long cystic duct remnant is higher than previously though. During common duct exploration or stone extractions in the postoperative period, calculi have been known to disappear into the spiral cystic duct stump (Fig. 4.17) (23, 24, 25).

The low insertion of the distal CBD in the second or third portion of the duodenum is not uncommon (Fig. 4.18), and it is very important to know before operative biliary endoscopy (cholangioscopy) is performed (for details see Chapter 5 Operative Biliary Endoscopy).

12. Cholecysto-Cholangiogram

In emergency cases the patients are often critically ill and the surgeon finds an extensive inflammatory, edematous process in the subhepatic region. Under these circumstances dissection can be difficult, and it may be risky to attempt isolation of the cystic duct for cannulation if the situation is not clear.

In these patients a suitable catheter or needle may be inserted into the gallbladder and after bile cultures are taken and the gallbladder emptied, contrast material may be injected (Fig. 4.19a). Because of the volume of the gallbladder, additional contrast material is usually required and should be available. A distended gallbladder frequently overlies the common bile duct, therefore, a rotation to the right to obtain maximum obliquity of the patient is nearly always necessary. Knowing the details of the ductal anatomy and the status of the common bile duct (stones?, sphincter function and appearance?) will allow progress of appropriate surgery in these high risk patients (Fig. 4.19b). A similar situation can also occur in elective cases wherein the patient has undergone previous gastric, right colon, or other upper abdominal surgery and firm adhesions make the dissection of the Calot triangle difficult and time consuming.

13. The choledocho-cholangiogram

Re-exploration in the cholecystectomized patient always present a challenge to the surgeon. Even if the location of the obstruction or calculus is preoperatively established by percutaneous transhepatic cholangiography or endoscopic retrograde cholangiography, the distortion of the anatomy due to adhesions of other organs to the right lobe of the liver can add time and difficulty to the dissection. It may be advisable to probe the area with a fine gauge needle attached to a syringe in an attempt to aspirate bile and establish the location of the duct. In those patients who underwent preoperative transhepatic biliary drainage with the catheter placed in the CBD, palpation of the indwelling catheter is helpful in identifying the duct.

As with primary biliary surgery, a cholangiogram performed early in the course of the secondary operation is important for demonstration of the anatomy and pathology. It also serves as a base-line with which the completion cholangiogram with its artifacts (postexploratory debris, air bubbles, etc.)

can be compared. If the results remain questionable, operative cholangioscopy has to be performed (or repeated) to resolve the dilemma.

Once the CBD is identified, various methods of cannulation have been used:

13.1. Direct needle puncture
A long needle attached directly to a syringe containing contrast material is inserted and two to three films are taken between injections. When the surgeon releases the syringe to step back during the exposure, the needle is easily dislodged.

13.2. Butterfly needle puncture
A 19 gauge butterfly needle with its attached extension tube may be employed (Fig. 4.20). The advantage is that the surgeon is at a distance from the X-ray beam during the exposures. Both techniques can suffer by inadvertent leakage of contrast material from the puncture site which can interfere with the interpretation of the findings.

13.3. Special needle clamp
Abbott employed a Babcock clamp to one limb of which a 21 gauge needle was soldered (Figs. 4.21a–b). With the clamp opened, the needle was inserted into the CBD. Closing the clamp grasped a portion of the duct fixing the position of the needle as well as preventing leakage. A previously attached extension tube allows the surgeon to inject from a distance (26). We modified this clamp to be able to replace the needle which can be easily damaged or broken during sterilization. A long curved hemostat can also be used. A hole in the horizontal limb can be drilled which will accomodate *a disposable needle*. It then functions like a modified Abbott clamp. Extravasation with this cannulation technique can be avoided (27).

The principles of fluorocholangiography as described for the cystic duct cholangiogram are then applied for the choledocho-cholangiogram. Controlled injection with attention to the early filling stage is emphasized.

13.4. T-tube insertion
After a choledochotomy (or choledocholithotomy) a large T-tube, Fr. 14 or greater, should be inserted and brought out to the flank in a relatively straight line in the event that postoperative intervention

through the T-tube tract becomes necessary. The recently available Whelan-Moss* T-tube facilitates this procedure.

14. Contact selective cholangiography

This technique which was largely developed by Yvergneaux (28, 29) provides excellent radiographic imaging of the sphincteric region of the CBD. Although not considered necessary in the majority of primary biliary operations, it is invaluable in the operative documentation of papillary stenosis in patients undergoing secondary biliary surgery for persistent symptoms after cholecystectomy, where it is used in conjunction with biliary manometry.

The procedure entails a preliminary mobilization of the duodenum and head of the pancreas. A sterile dental X-ray film is then inserted behind the lower end of the bile duct and head of the pancreas. Filling of the bile duct with contrast is either with gravity feed or slow pump infusion. A KV of 80,is used with an exposure of 300 mA in apnoea. If a terminal stricture and dilated CBD are documented, the contact selective cholangiogram is repeated after intravenous administration of either CCK or Ceruletide. If the narrowing persists, organic stenosis is confirmed. Figs. 4.22a–b, 4.23a–b. The pressure changes in benign papillary stenosis are dealt with in Chapter 6.

15. Reason for failure of operative cholangiography

15.9. Overfilled ducts
When the injected contrast material is too concentrated (50–60%) or a large volume is injected small calculi can be easily obscured.

15.2. Underfilled ducts
Failure to visualize the entire biliary system may occur when too little contrast material is injected or when a flaccid sphincter allows immediate free drainage into duodenum. In this situation the hepatic branches, particularly the left which courses anteriorly, are inadequately displayed.

*Davol Co., Rhode Island, U.S.A.

15.2. Poor quality films
Suboptimal imaging may be due to inadequate techniques such as insufficient beam penetration particularly in the obese subject, poor contrast, or unsharpness due to long exposures.

15.4. Improper positioning
If the patient is not rotated as described above, the distal CBD may be over-shadowed by the spine. Some areas of the anatomy (sphincter or hepatic branches) can be missed or are not in the field at all.

15.5. Obscured field
The CBD may be obscured by instruments or radio-opaque material left in the wound, such as surgical clips and sponges, NG tubes, EKG leads, or remnants of barium in the hepatic flexure can also overlie the CBD.

16. Artifacts

In this setting, artifacts refer to radiolucent defects *not due to calculi*, which appear in the bile duct filled with contrast material. Unfortunately, these defects often simulate calculi and differentiation can be extremely difficult.

(a) Air bubbles are frequently seen if insufficient care was taken in rinsing the system or expulsion of air prior to injection. If air, despite these preventive measures, was injected the duct should be rinsed with saline to clear the bubbles and contrast material and the cholangiogram should be repeated. Bubbles may also be confirmed fluoroscopically by the rapid to and from movement with the syringe plunger creating alternating positive and negative pressure causing visible movements of these round lucencies synchronous with the syringe plunger action.

(b) External compression of the common bile duct by the traversing hepatic aretery can produce a thin transverse radiolucency (Fig. 4.24).

(c) Hemobilia may result in one or more thrombi which cannot be distinguished from calculi. A single ovoid or elongated filling defect may suggest a thrombus (Fig. 4.25).

(d) Cholangitis produces pus or desquamative debris which may aggregate and mimic calculi.

Similar defects are *very frequently* seen on completion cholangiograms after repeated or prolonged manipulations in the lumen of the ductal system following stone extraction attempts (Fig. 4.26a–d).

(e) Sphincter spasm preventing contrast material from entering the duodenum may occur particularly after *prolonged manipulation and passing instruments through the sphincter*. If fluoro-cholangiography is employed observations of the sphincter for a minute or two during slight positive injection pressure will usually allow the operator to witness a cycle of sphincter contraction and relaxation. To wait for a short period of time and re-fluoroscope the patient can also given information about the changes in sphincter configuration and show the appearance of contrast material in the duodenum (Fig. 4.27a–d and 4.27e–g). If these maneuvers are unsuccessful, cholangioscopy may be necessary.

17. Complications of operative cholangiography

Complications are extremely rare and are usually due to either hypersensitivity to contrast material or excessive injection pressure. Patients with documented previous idiosyncrasy to contrast material are at a risk from operative cholangiography using iodinated contrast agents. For these patients a suspension of pre-sterilized barium powder and sterile saline in appropriate ratio, provides a satisfactory contrast medium. We use a mixture of 30 cc of Barosperse® and 90 cc of water (Fig. 4.28). Rinsing the duct with saline following cholangiography helps to clear the barium.

Excessive injection pressure can result in bacteremia and bile duct rupture. Bacteremia is even more likely in the patient with an established cholangitis (30).

Elevated intraductal pressures forces micro ruptures of bile canaliculi and can provide bacterial access to the circulation. Occasionally a ductal rupture will be manifest by a hepatic parenchymal stain of contrast material (Fig. 4.5).

18. Reformed calculi

The origin of common duct stones presenting years after a cholecystectomy remains controversial (31, 32). For instance, were these calculi missed at the original operation or have they formed de novo? Stones which arise de novo within the CBD are usually soft and fragment easily and may be simply a compaction of biliary sludge or mud. Lithogenic bile and stasis as occurs in ampullary stenosis or partial obstruction of other etiology, are also contributory factors in some cases.

An example of reformed stones is seen in the case of a 60 year old Caucasian male who underwent cholecystectomy. Initial cystic duct cholangiography displayed stones in the CBD (Fig. 4.29). Choledocholithotomy was performed and the stones were removed. A negative completion cholangiogram was obtained at the end of the procedure. In the immediate postoperative period another T-tube cholangiogram was made (Fig. 4.29b) which displayed a small duct, free of calculi and without outflow obstruction. Two years later he was admitted with abdominal pain, chills, and jaundice. Endoscopic retrograde cholangiography displayed a dilated duct with calculi in both the CBD and the cystic duct remnant (Fig. 4.29c–d). A successful endoscopic sphincterotomy was performed which was followed by spontaneous passage of stones and reduction in the caliber of the CBD (Fig. 4.29e).

In our opinion no calculi were missed at the initial operation nor did a sphincter stenosis or outflow obstruction exist. These calculi reformed within two years. Bile analysis was not performed.

19. Complications of T-tube removal in the postoperative period

In our series of 260 CBD explorations with T-tube drainage, complications occurred after pulling the T-tube in three patients (1.1%). In all these cases the postoperative T-tube cholangiogram was normal with no outflow obstruction or retained calculi observed. The cholangiogram was performed on the seventh to ninth postoperative day, and the tubes were pulled after this event on the 9th to 21st day.

Case 1: 60 year old male developed sudden abdominal pain immediately following the T-tube removal which evolved into an acute abdomen within the next few hours. Emergency laparotomy revealed bile accumulation in the right peritoneal gutter and no sinus tract formation was found between the CBD and the right flank. Bile leaked freely from the opening of the CBD. A catheter was placed through the opening into the CBD and left in position for another two months. The patient had an uneventful postoperative course. When the tube was pulled 8 weeks after the second intervention no further complication occurred. The patient had a history of diabetes which was under control

Case 2: 72 year old Caucasian female who underwent cholecystectomy for classical symptoms of cholelithiasis. Initial cystic cholangiography displayed a calculus in the distal CBD and choledocholithotomy with a negative completion T-tube cholangiogram was performed. The patient had an uneventful course and a negative postoperative T-tube cholangiogram was performed on the eighth postoperative day. The tube was pulled on the following day. The patient complained of abdominal pain and tenderness during the next 24 h and an ultrasound scan showed fluid accumulation in the right subphrenic space. The fluid was aspirated under CT guidance and proved to be bile. A pigtail catheter was inserted percutaneously for drainage. The patient's general condition improved, and the drainage ceased within one week. The drainage catheter was withdrawn and the patient discharged.

Case 3: 53 year old white female who was on a steroid regimen because of a long standing rheumatoid arthritis. The patient underwent choledocholithotomy. The completion cholangiogram and the postoperative T-tube cholangiogram were negative. Because of her underlying disease her tube was pulled 4 weeks after the last T-tube X-rays. She developed immediately, abdominal symptoms requiring exploration. Bile accumulation with an incompletely formed sinus tract was found. A tube was replaced into the CBD. The patient

had an uneventful postoperative recovery. The tube was removed 2 months later after X-ray control.

An adequate tract of connective tissue formation is assumed to surround the T-tube after 7 to 10 days, but under certain circumstances this may not be the case. When postoperative removal of retained stones is necessary, the tract is given 6 weeks to mature. If only thin, filmy tissues have developed around the T-tube, they may be easily disrupted by the traumatic T-tube withdrawal. During pulling the tube the horizontal limb doubles on itself and the tract, which was formed around the tube, must now accomodate both horizontal limbs. Notching the horizontal limb of the T-tube opposite the vertical limb or complete removal of the opposite wall prior to its insertion effectively reduces the mass of the tube being pulled through the tract, thus diminishing the effect of trauma. The tract is apparently most tenuous at its junction with the CBD or abdominal wall.

It may be safer, therefore, to allow the T-tube to remain for a longer period of time prior to its withdrawal, especially in those patients where wound healing may be impaired as in the diabetic, severe arteriosclerotic, malnourished or the immuno-supressed. In these patients, withdrawal of the tube under fluoroscopic control accompanied by injection of contrast material prior to its complete removal will assess the integrity of the tract. If a leak occurs the radiologist can introduce a guide wire through the T-tube and sinus tract back into the CBD. The T-tube can then be completely withdrawn and another tube (drainage) inserted coaxially over the guide wire into the extrahepatic biliary system. This will prevent bile leakage and its serious sequelae.

In our opinion, leakage occurs more frequently than clinical symptoms would indicate (33). The subclinical picture of leakage is probably present in more than half of the cases. It is difficult to believe that the connective tissue sinus tract can be formed from the the CBD to the parietal peritoneum in 8 to 10 days. As an analogy, the high incidence of subclinical leakage in low rectal anastomosis without severe symptoms is well documented.

We urge, therefore, that this complication be kept in mind before pulling the T-tube. It should not be removed prematurely. The T-tube horizontal limb should be kept short or cut in half. In those cases where a delay in the healing proces is anticipated due to the various factors mentioned above, a clamped T-tube should be kept for a longer period of time and the pulling procedure should be performed by a radiologist under fluoroscopic-radiographic control.

20. Results of operative cholangiography

The majority of publications evaluate only completion T-tube cholangiograms performed at the end of the exploration. This procedure harbors a much greater incidence of false-positive and/or false-negative results than an initial cholangiogram as mentioned in paragraph 5 of this chapter. Therefore, in assessing operative cholangiography, two groups should be separated:

    (a) initial and

    (b) completion cholangiography.

In our first report of fluoro-cholangiography, out of 556 consecutive cases, 447 were cystic duct cholangiograms. We had one false-negative and two-false positive cases (0.6%) resulting in a diagnostic accuracy of 99.4%.

In the completion T-tube group of 119 cases, we had 4 false-negatives (3.3%) concluding in a 96.7% diagnostic accuracy (19).

In the following three years we accumulated a further experience of additional 909 cholangiograms out of which 191 were CBD explorations.

In the group of 718 cystic duct cholangiograms, our reading error remained the same (4/718 = 0.55%), but in the group of completion T-tube cholangiograms, our failure rate increased slightly from the previous 3.3% to 6%. This was partially due to human factors that, despite the radiologist declaring the appearance as a cholangitis, the surgeon explored the duct because of the patient's history, presence of jaundice or if the radiologist was not quite sure and not insistent enough to ask for a repeat and the duct was opened.

There is another reason why we prefer the initial cholangiograms where the interpretative error is less. In 11% of all biliary cases (mainly simple or elective cholecystectomies) a cholangiogram was not performed due to obstruction or extremely narrow cystic duct and the patient had no symptoms or biochemical evidence of a ductal obstruction. In these cases the surgeons were not inclined to add a puncture wound of the CBD to perform a choledocho-cholangiogram. In 90% of all CBD explorations operative biliary endoscopy was performed and the bottom line is that the incidence of retained stones in the group of 191 CBD explorations was only 3.6%. It is a significant decrease from our previous results (See Chapter 5 Operative Biliary Endoscopy).

Having an experience of seven years using fluoro-cholangiography with serial film techniques (6 to 12 films per patient) exposed during fluoroscopy, our surgical staff members were convinced about the superiority and efficiency of this equipment. The advantages of the technique overshadow the disadvantages.

20.1. Advantages

The diagnostic accuracy is greater because *serial films* provide the radiologist and surgeons with a greater safety margin for evaluation with a high and uniform film quality. The equipment can be shared with other specialties (orthopedic, urologic, thoracic surgery, etc.) which today requires intraoperative radiology as well, and therefore, it became as improved interdisciplinary modality. Another important factor is the utilization of the operating rooms. In our experience we saved 20 min per biliary case employing fixed, installed equipment vs. the portable machines. This accumulates (per annum) in an institution with sizeable biliary material, and increases the number of cases operated upon within the same time period.

20.2. Disadvantages

It requires well trained technicians because the equipment is more complex. The investment is approximately 3 to 4 times more than a portable unit.

But the advantages far outweigh the disadvantages from the point of improved patient care and the economics. If we are considering the cost effectiveness of cholangiography, we should always compare the best available techniques and not the obsolete ones. Furthermore, not very much has been said about the expenses involved with a missed stone. Table 4.1 displays the real cost expressed in time and personnel required for removal of re-

Table 4.1

	1		2		3	4	5	6
Procedure	Procedure room	No. of hrs.	Personnel utilized	No. of hrs.	Instrument deprec.	Disposable items	Hospital iz. days	Professional fees
Stone extraction	+	1	O.R. technician	1	++	+	out-patient	Radiologist
			X-ray technician	1				Surgeon
			R.N.	1				
Perfusion	+ (X-ray)	2–3	X-ray technician	2–3	+	++	7–10	Radiologist
								Physician
Endoscopic papillotomy	+	1	R.N.	1	++	+	4–5	Endoscopist
			G.I. technician	1				
Follow-up ERC post papillotomy	+	1/2	R.N.	1/2	++	+		
			G.I. technician	1/2				
Re-exploration	++ (O.R.)	3–4	Included in O.R. fees	–	+	++	8–10	Surgeon
								Assistants
								Anes-thesiolog.

Hospital charges 1–5
Professional fees 6
+ = >$200
++ = <$200

tained stones using various modalities. Every type of health delivery care system can substitute their own figures in this table and get some idea about the actual expenses. In this assessment the patient's loss, being out of work for several months and the deficit to the society in form of a decreased labor force, is not included. If we are taking all of these aspects into consideration, then this slight increase of capital outlay for larger institutions is very worthwhile to consider.

References

1. Mirizzi PL: La Cholangiografia durante las Operaciones de las vias Biliares. Bol Soc Cir Buenos Aires 16:1133–1161, 1932.
2. Mirizzi PL: Operative cholangiography. Surg Gynecol & Obstet, 65:702–709, 1937.
3. Hicken NF, McAllister AJ, Franz B, Crowder F: Technique, indications and value of postoperative cholangiography. Arch Surg 50:1102–1113, 1950.
4. Hicken NF, Best RR, Hunt HB: Cholangiography. Ann Surg 103:210–229, 1936.
5. Hess W: Operative cholangiographie. Stuttgart, Thieme, 1965.
6. Nottle PD, Hughes ESR, McDermott FT: Cholecystectomy without routine operative cholangiography. Aust N Z J Surg 52:484–487, 1982.
7. Skillings JC, Williams JS, Hinshaw JR: Cost-effectiveness of operative cholangiography. AM J Surg 137:26–31, 1979.
8. Deitch EA, Voci VE: Operative cholangiography: The case for selective instead of routine operative cholangiography. Amer Surg 48:297–301, 1982.
9. Chant ADB, Dewbury KG, Guyer PB, Goh H: Operative cholangiography reassessed. Clin Radiol 33:289–291, 1982.
10. Schein CJ, Stern WZ, Jacobson HG: The common bile duct. Springfield, Charles C. Thomas, 1966.
11. Bartlett MK, Wadell WR: Indications for common duct exploration N Engl J Med 258:164–168, 1958.
12. Farha GJ, Pearson RN: Transcystic duct operative cholangiography. Am J Surg 131:228–231, 1975.

32

13. Chatterjee DK, Jones WM: Value of operative cholangiography. Brit J Surg 32:105–106, 1978.
14. Berci G, Hamlin JA: Unsuspected Stone(s) In: Operative Biliary Radiology. Berci G, Hamlin JA (eds), Baltimore, Williams & Wilkins, 1982, p 137–139.
15. Shore JM, Berci G: A simple rapid technique for cystic duct cholangiography. Am J Surg 123:741–742, 1972.
16. Berci G, Shore JM: Improved cannula for operative (cystic duct) cholangiography. Am J Surg 137:826–828, 1979.
17. Borge J: Operative cholangiography. Arch Surg 112:340–342, 1977.
18. Feeley M, Peel ALG: A critical assessment of fluoroscopy in peroperative cholangiography. Ann Roy Coll Surg 64:180–182, 1982.
19. Hamlin JA, Berci G: The fluoro-cholangiogram. In: Operative Biliary Radiology. Berci G, Hamlin JA (eds), Baltimore, Williams & Wilkins, 1982, p 63–109.
20. Hamlin JA, Berci G: Technique. In: Operative Biliary Radiology. Berci G, Hamlin JA (eds), Baltimore, Williams & Wilkins, 1982, p 68.
21. Hamlin JA: Biliary ductal anomalies. In: Operative Biliary Radiology. Berci G, Hamlin JA (eds), Baltimore, Williams & Wilkins, 1982, p 109–137.
22. Early D: Radiation hazard. In: Operative Biliary Radiology. Berci G, Hamlin JA (eds), Baltimore, Williams & Wilkins, 1982, p 27–55.
23. Ruge E: Beitrage zur chirurgischen Anatomie der grossen Gallenwege. Arch Klin Chir 87:47–53, 1908.
24. Wiechel KL: Surgical anatomy of bile ducts: The cystic duct. In: Operative Biliary Radiology. Berci G, Hamlin JA (es), Baltimore, Williams & Wilkins, 1982, p 37–50.
25. Hamlin JA: Biliary Ductal Anomalies: The cystic duct. In: Operative Biliary Radiology. Berci G, Hamlin JA (eds), Baltimore, Williams & Wilkins, 1982, p 120–126.
26. Abbott CA: A new instrument for operative cholangiography. Surg Gynecol Obstet 119:854–856, 1964.
27. Berci G, Hamlin JA: Re-exploration. The Choledocho-cholangiogram: Cannulation technique. In: Operative Biliary Radiology. Berci G, Hamlin JA (eds), Baltimore, Williams & Wilkins, 1982, p 160–161.
28. Yvergneaux JP: Apport du cliche Intra-abdominal au Diagnostic de la Stenose Oddienne Benigne. Acta Gastroenterol Belgica 32:407– , 1969.
29. Yvergneaux JP, Bauwens E, Van Outryve L, Yvergneaux E: Benign stenosis of the papilla of Vater. Acta Chir Belgica 76:523, 1977.
30. Schein CJ: Complications of operative cholangiography. In: The Common Bile Duct. Schein C, Stern WZ, Jacobson HG (eds), Springfield, Charles C. Thomas, 1966.
31. Madden JL, Vanderheyden L, Kandalaft S: The nature and surgical significance of common suct stones. Surg Gynecol & Obstet 126:2–8, 1968.
32. Saharia PC, Zuidema GD, Cameron JL: Primary common duct stones. Ann Surg 185:598–605, 1977.
33. Domeliof L, Rydh A, Truedson H: Leakage from T-tube tracts as determined by contrast radiology. Brit J Surg 64:862–863, 1977.

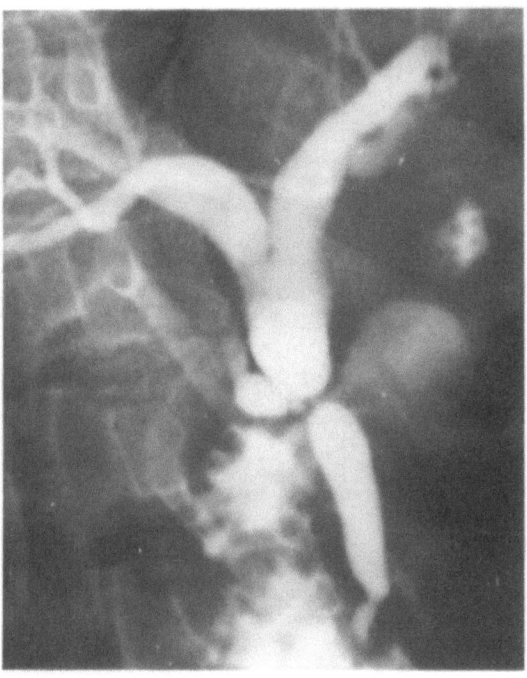

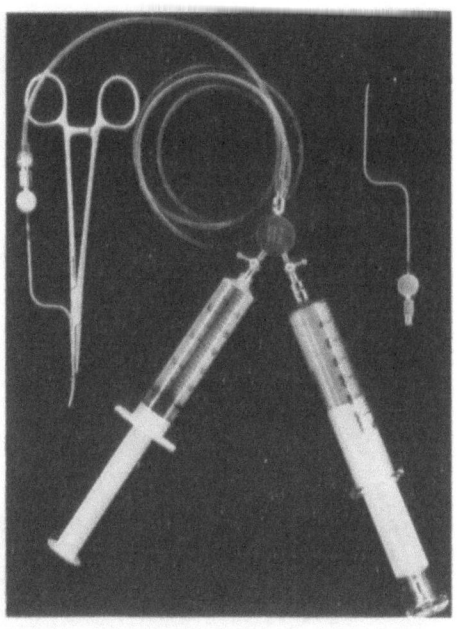

Fig. 4.1. Iatrogenic stricture. Recurrent bouts of cholangitis, beginning in the postoperative period following cholecystectomy four years earlier, led to a bilio-enteric bypass.

Fig. 4.2a. A metal cannula (outside diameters 1.5 and 2.0 mm) is connected to a double stopcock via a venous extension tube. A 20 cc plastic syringe with saline and a 30 cc glass syringe with contrast material. Squeeze lock clamp holding the smaller cannula. Air bubbles are carefully extruded.

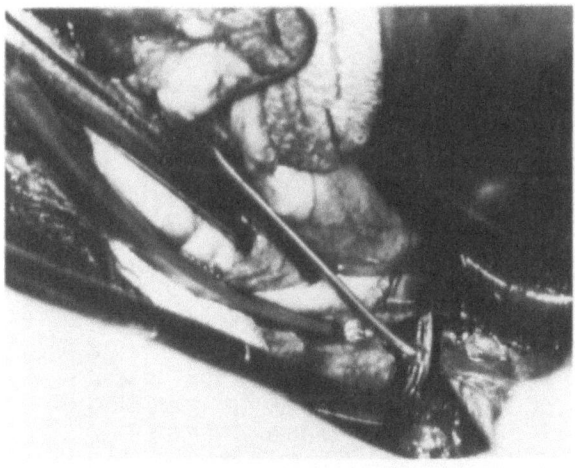

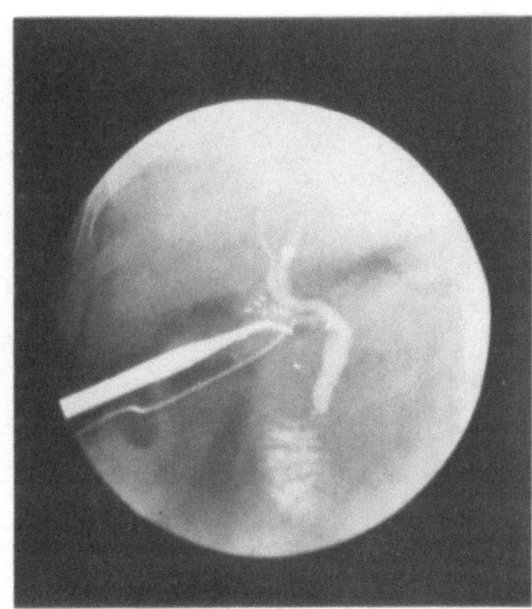

Fig. 4.2b. In obese patients it is easy to cannulate a small hole at a great depth without obscuring the vision. The assistant applies the cannula fixing clamp.

Fig. 4.2c. The radio-opaque cannula and its position are well seen on the X-ray film.

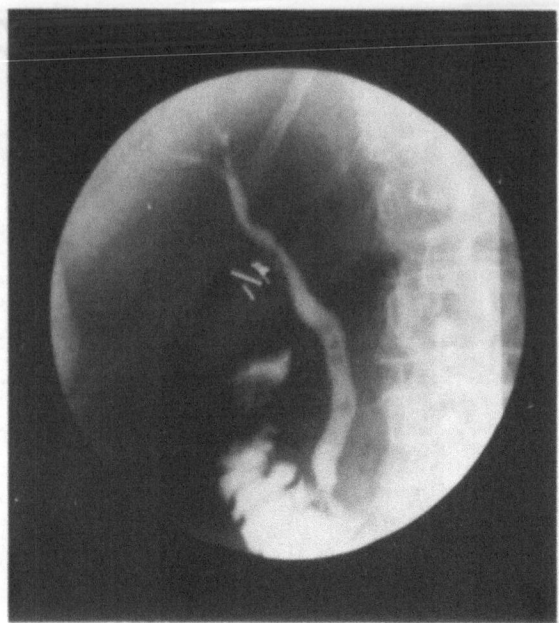

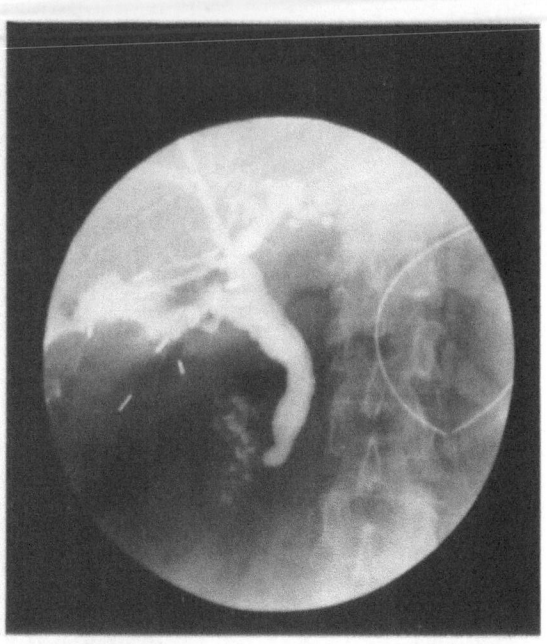

Fig. 4.2d. Air bubbles. Multiple round radiolucencies within the CBD. Often it is difficult to distinguish bubbles from calculi, and therefore, meticulous technique is required to prevent their introduction into the biliary tree.

Fig. 4.2e. Extravasation due to insufficient closure of the duct around cannula can result in overshadowing of the CBD, creating difficulty in evaluation.

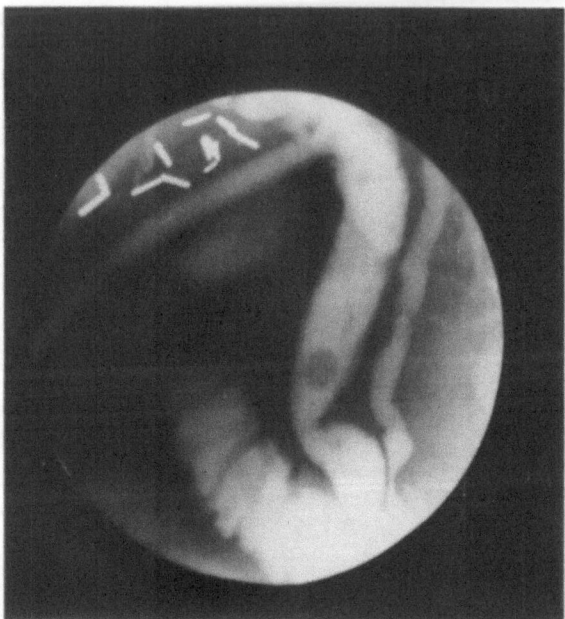

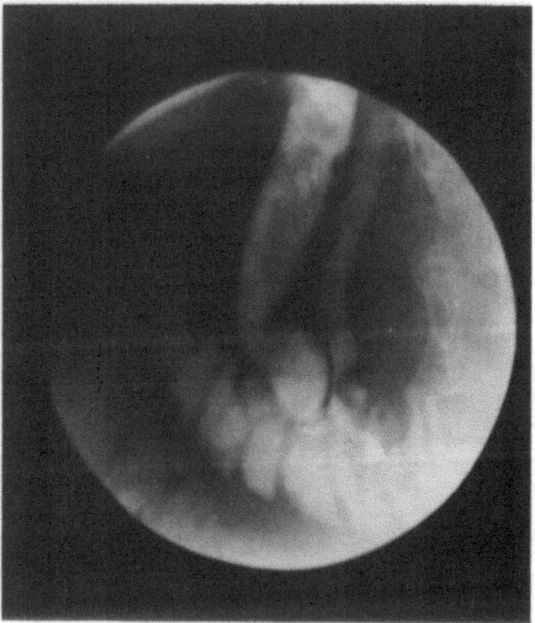

Fig. 4.3a. Air bubble on completion cholangiogram. Air commonly gains access to the CBD during duct exploration, and bubbles seen on the completion cholangiogram can simulate calculi. Rinsing the CBD with saline prior to cholangiography will clear it of bubbles. If a bubble persists, however, it may be identified fluoroscopically by its motion commensurate with the rapid injection-withdrawal movements of the syringe plunger.

Fig. 4.3b. After extended manipulation cholangitic debris and/or blood clots can mimic calculi. This case was interpreted as 'cholangitis.' In problematic situations biliary endoscopy can solve the dilemma.

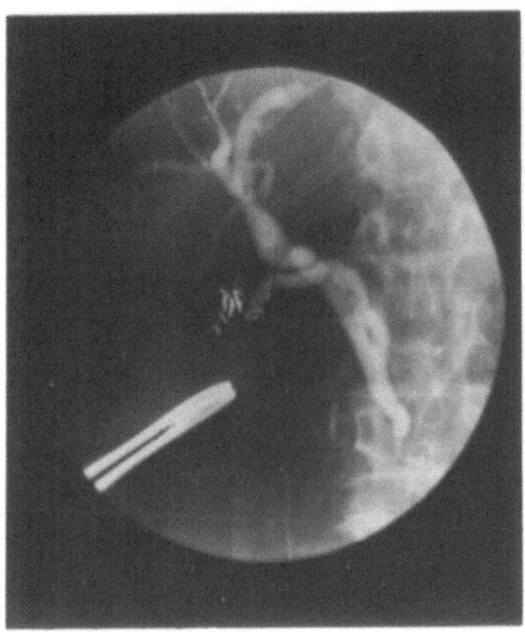

Fig. 4.4. If the patient is not rotated 10 to 15° to the right the CBD can be superimposed over the spine. Note the spiral course of the cystic duct stump.

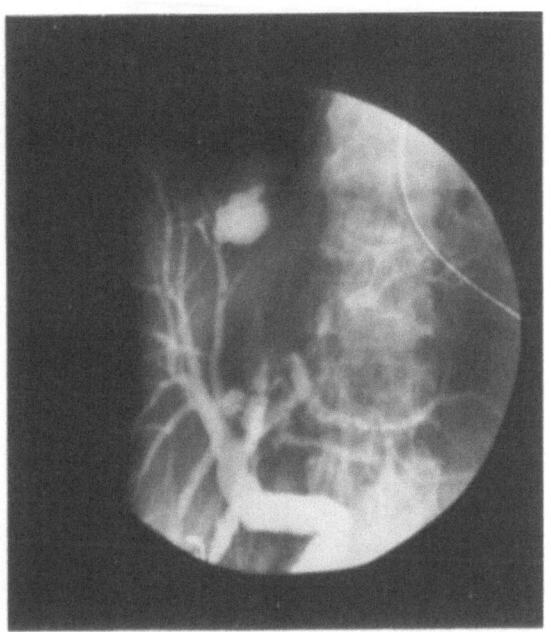

Fig. 4.5. Intra-hepatic extravasation. Excessive injection pressure can rupture small intra-hepatic branches. By fluoroscopically monitoring the injection overdistention can be prevented. A similar finding occurs with ductal rupture by an excessively inflated catheter balloon.

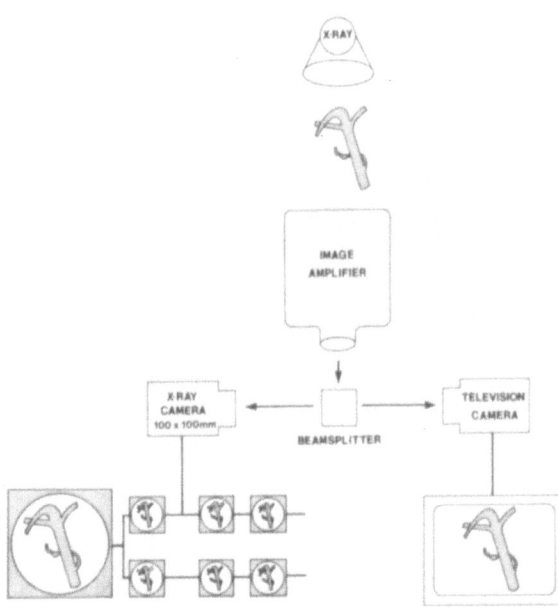

Fig. 4.6a. Schematic diagram of a modern video system. The visible image is directed via a rotating beam splitter from the image amplifier (IA) to a television camera and viewed on the TV monitor. By pressing a button (footswitch) the image is transferred to an X-ray camera loaded with 200, 100 × 100 mm (4 × 4 in) cut films. *Indirect radiography* refers to the photographic production of films from the output phosphor of the IA rather than by direct X-ray exposure.

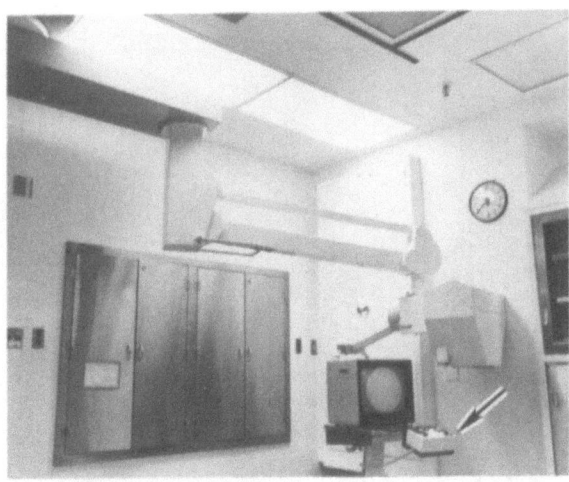

Fig. 4.6b. Overhead tube crane in parking position. No floor space is occupied. It can be moved in position much faster and more accurately than a portable machine. Remote control box with TV monitor on wheels (arrow). Tube output: 150 kV; focal spots: 0.6–1.2 mm with built-in automatic collimating system. Because of the larger energy output, shorter exposure times are required only (1/10–1/30th of a second).

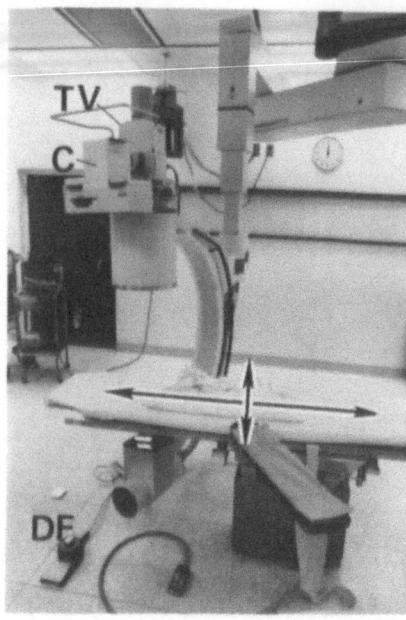

Fig. 4.6c. Ceiling suspended C-arm. The equipment and per-formance are the same as described in Figures 4.6a–b. This equipment has the advantage of providing oblique views by rotating the C-arm rather than the patient. Surgical tabletop with coordinate movements (arrows). DF = double footswitch for fluoroscopy and radiography. Alignment is provided by a fixed C-arm connection.

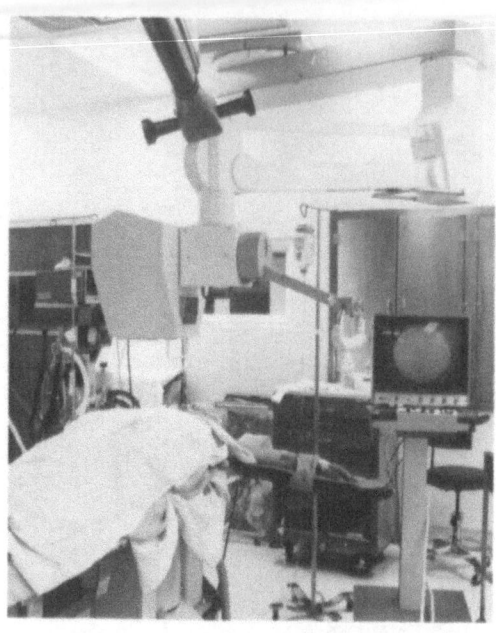

Fig. 4.6d. Patient prepared for scout film. Tube in position. Monitor at patient's left. Scout films are exposed before anes-thesia is induced and scrutinized by the X-ray technician and surgeon for proper positioning and exposure technique.

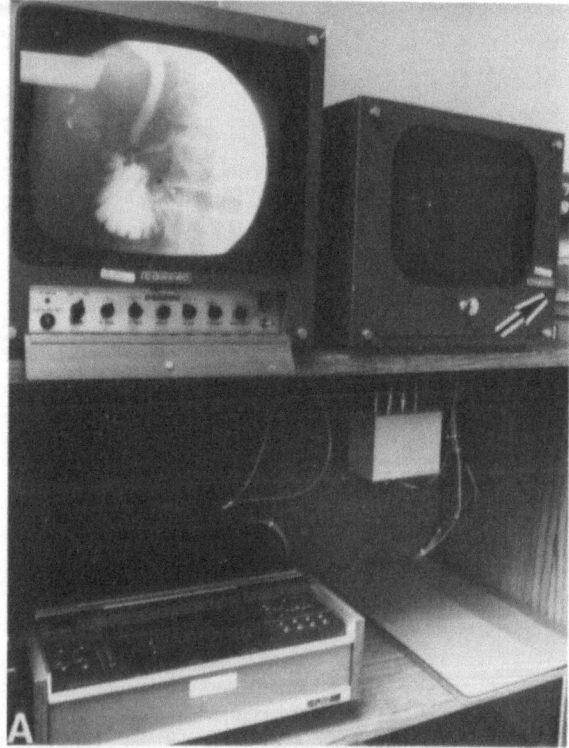

Fig. 4.6e. Audio (arrow) and visual intercom system between the operating rooms and X-ray department. The radiologist can observe the fluoroscopic appearance and direct the entire pro-cedure. Video-tape (3/4 in. cassette) is placed below the TV monitor.

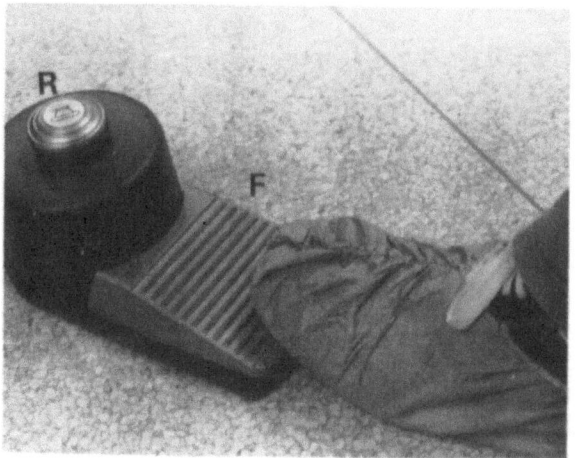

Fig. 4.6f. The most convenient and important accessory for the surgeon: the double footswitch. F = fluoroscopy. Only short exposures are employed. At the appropriate phase of contrast material injection, the switch R (radiography) is pressed and a 100 × 100 mm film is automatically exposed and the next film is placed into the gate of the camera. Switching back and forth between fluoroscopy and radiography is done quickly. There is no need to lift drapes or replace cassettes. In 5 to 6 min the entire cholangiographic process including positioning of the machine, slow injection, fluoroscopy and exposures of 12 films can be completed.

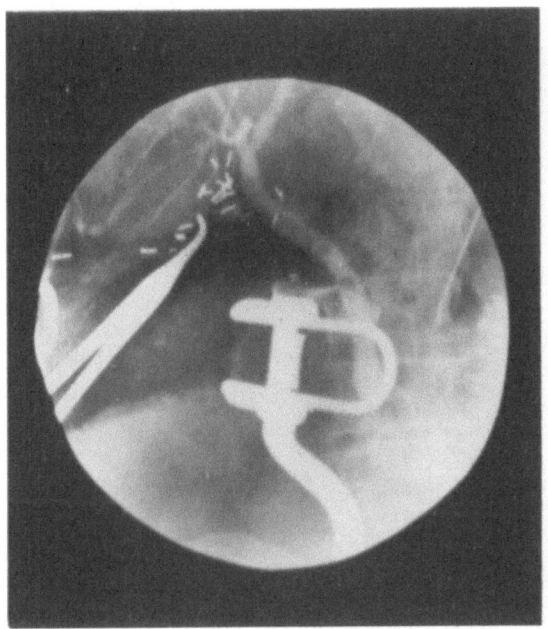

Fig. 4.7a. Retractor left in a position overlapping the distal duct.

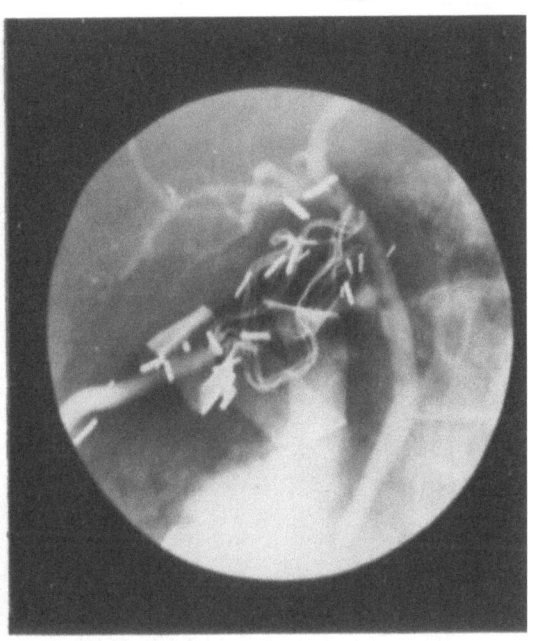

Fig. 4.7b. Sponges with radio-opaque markers were inadvertently left in the field during cholangiography.

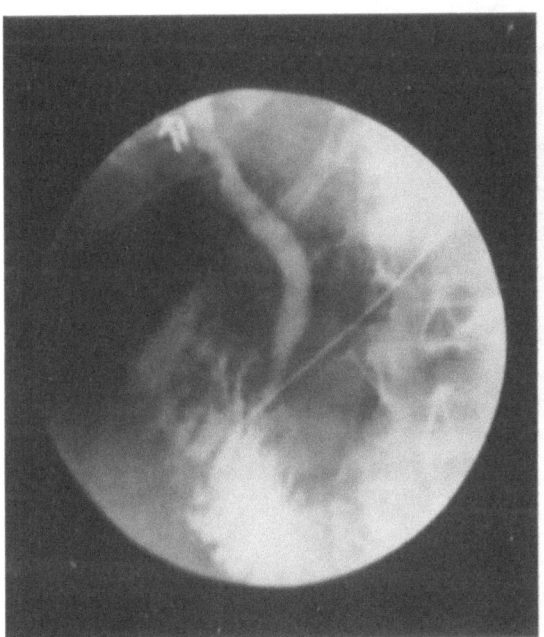

Fig. 4.7c. Naso-gastric tube with radio-opaque marker crossing the ampullary region. The anesthesiologist should be asked to withdraw it into the proximal stomach.

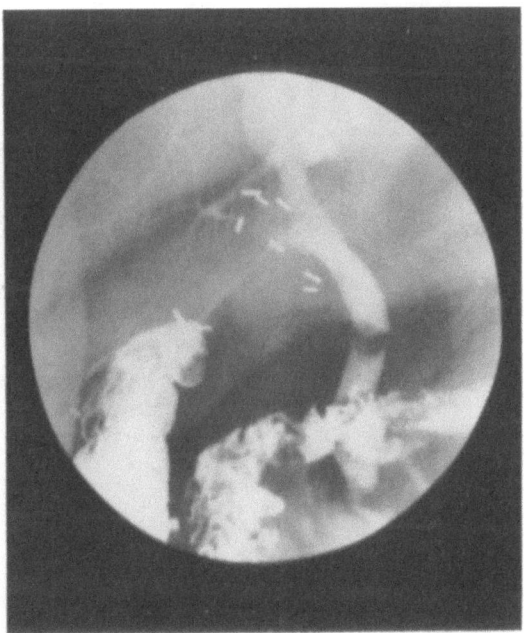

Fig. 4.7d. A preoperative upper gastrointestinal or barium enema examination may result in a hepatic flexure filled with barium which could obscure the distal CBD. A scout film the day prior to surgery is useful to determine if additional colon cleansing is necessary.

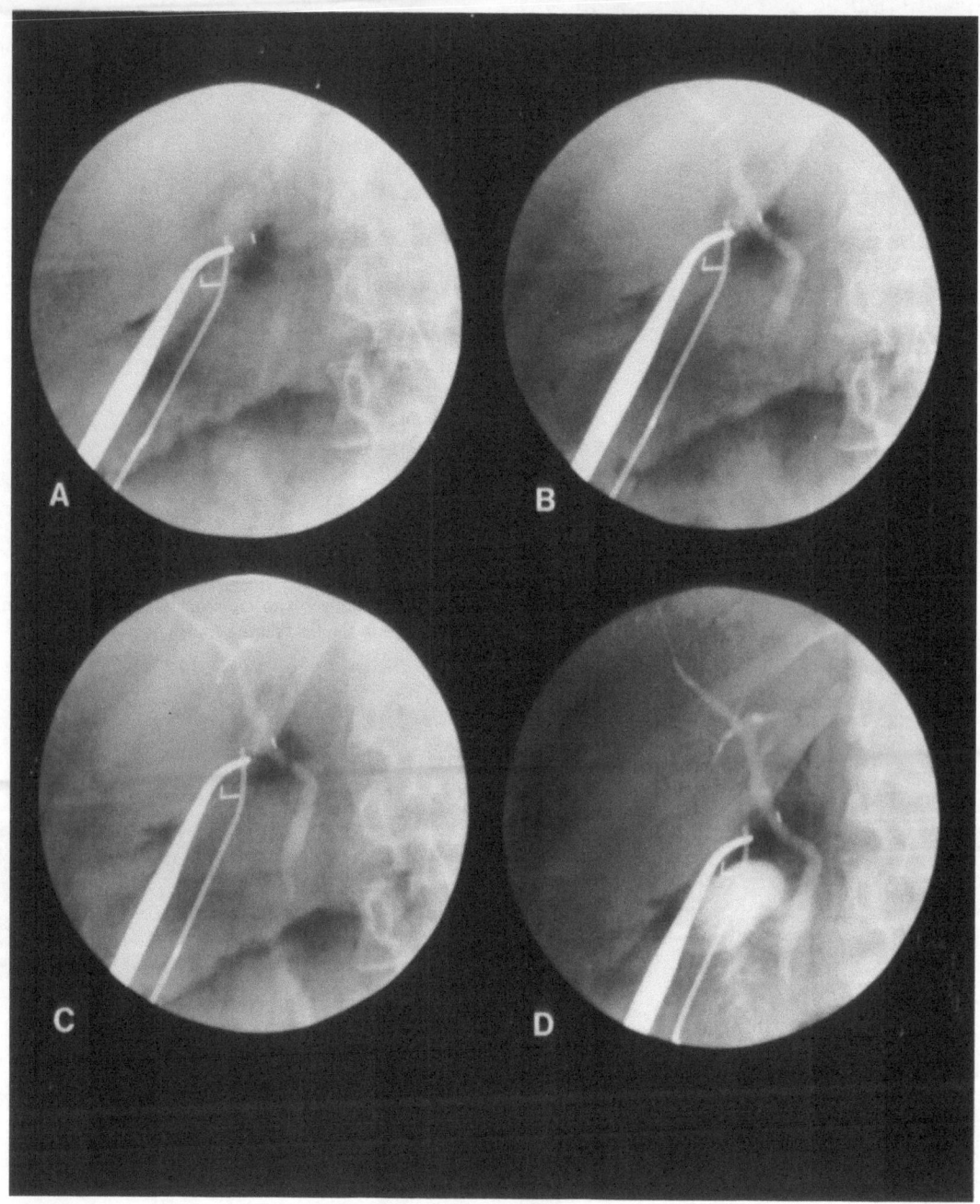

Figs. 4.8a–h. Serial film technique. At the first appearance of contrast material entering the ductal system as observed on the television screen, a film is taken. Subsequent films are exposed after each 1–2 ml of injection. Using this technique we can be sure that the extra-intra-hepatic biliary system is filled gradually without running the risk of obscuring smaller calculi with excessive contrast material. Overfilling is the case in the majority of cholangiograms performed 'blindly' with the standard technique. By pressing a button, electronic enlargement can be achieved, switching from a 10 in to a 6 in input screen (see picture e and h) and greater detail can be observed.

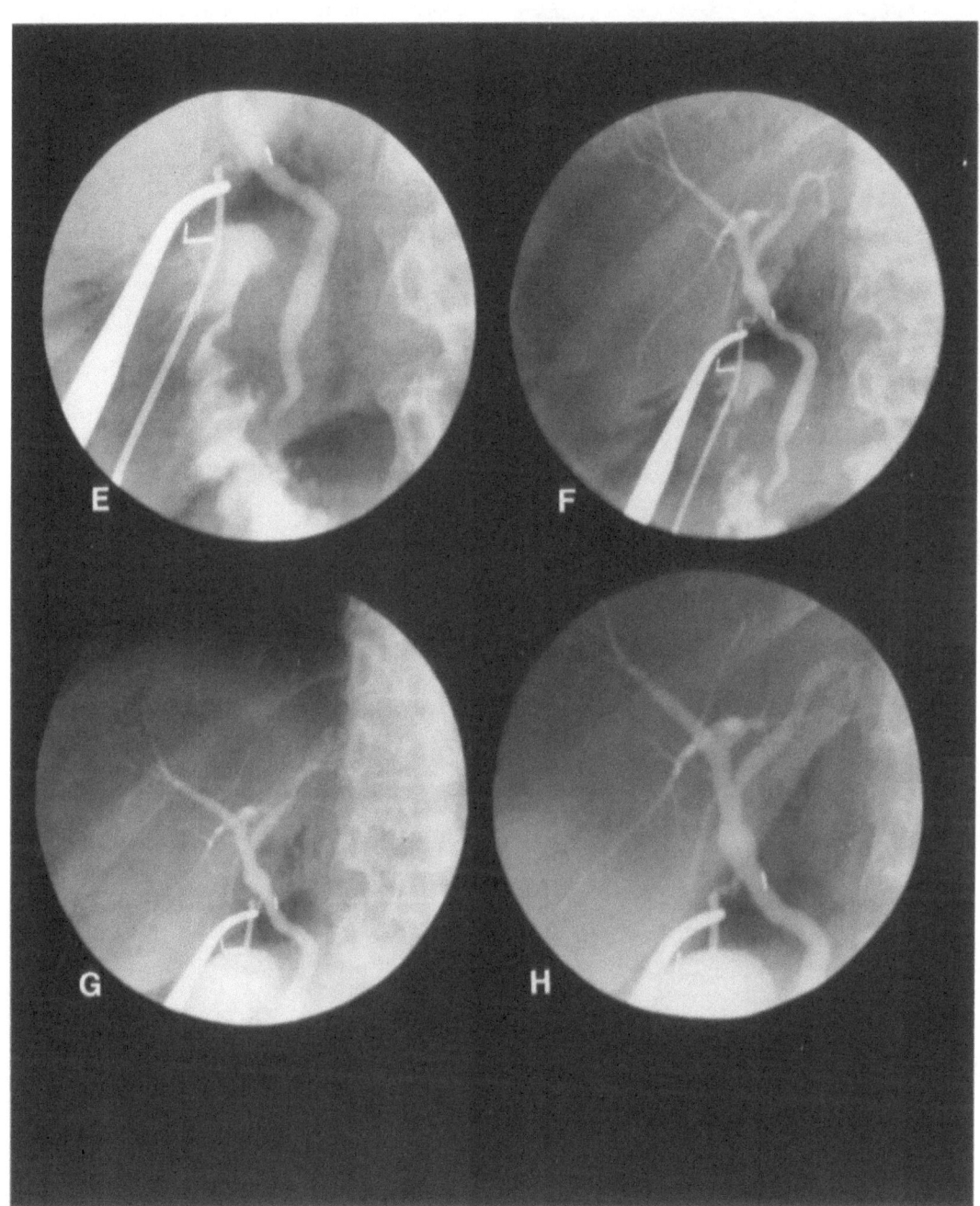

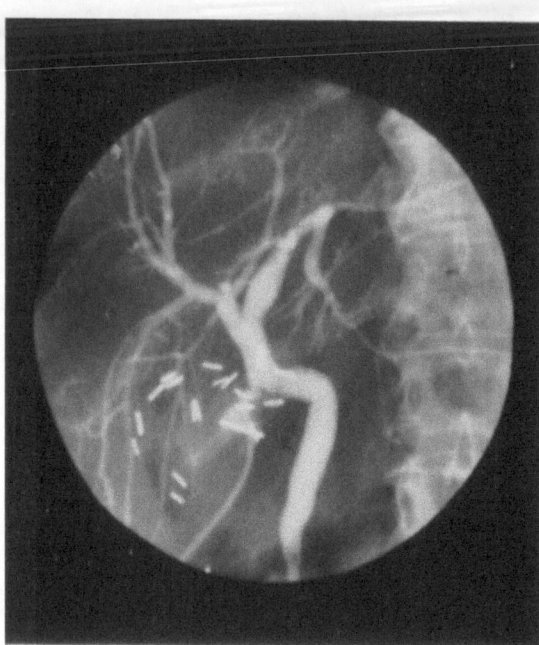

Fig. 4.9. Branches as small as 1–2 mm in diameter can be displayed. The resolution of an indirect radiograph for cholangiography is more than sufficient. Note the small calculus in the distal duct.

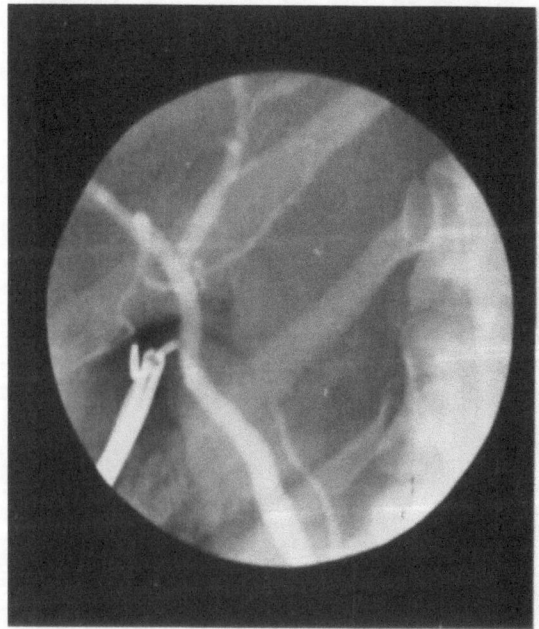

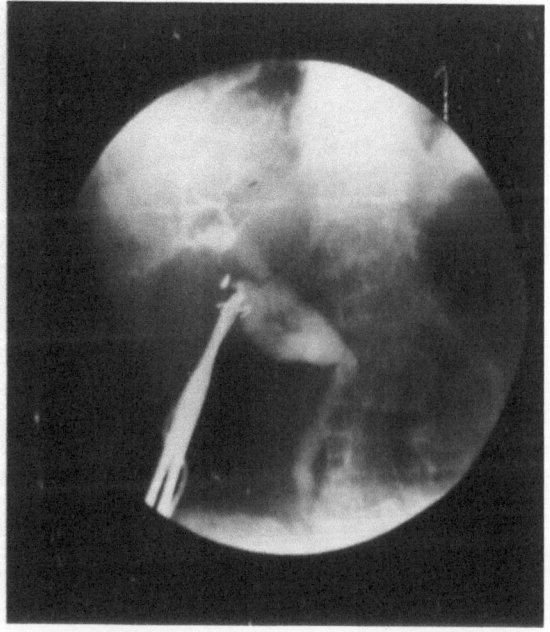

Fig. 4.10a. Display of a short cystic duct can warn the surgeon to ligate the stump carefully without impinging or severing the common duct.

Fig. 4.10b. Dilated cystic duct entering posteriorly into the CBD. Without cholangiography this cystic duct could be mistaken for the common duct.

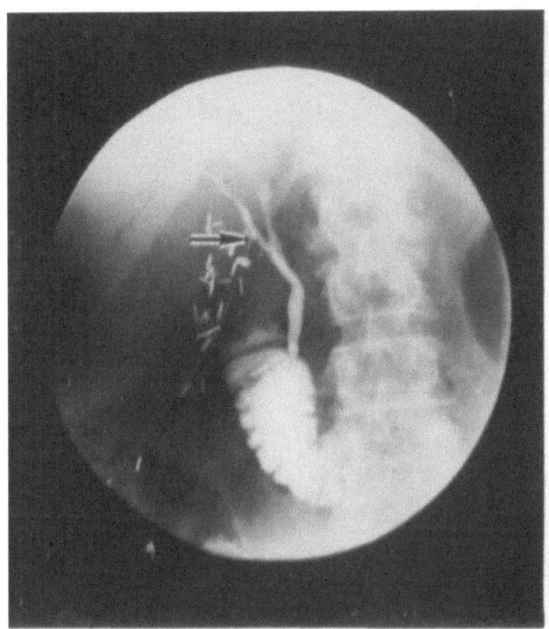

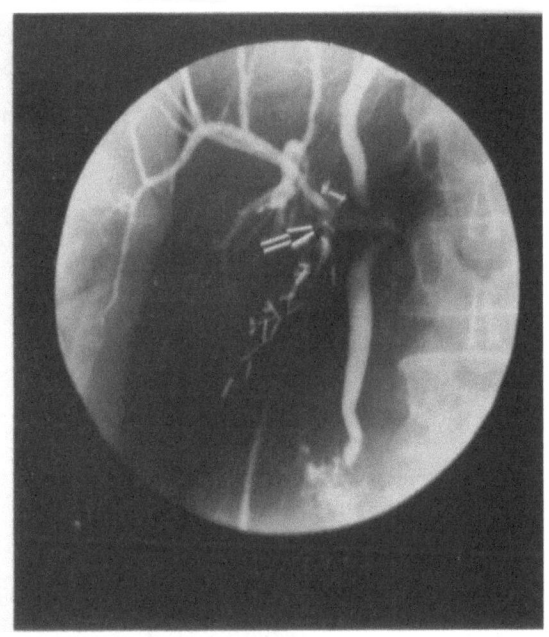

Fig. 4.11a. Cystic duct drainage into a right hepatic branch. Recognition of this anomaly early in the dissection is critical.

Fig. 4.11b. Cystic duct entering the right hepatic duct which then joins the CBD in a spiral course.

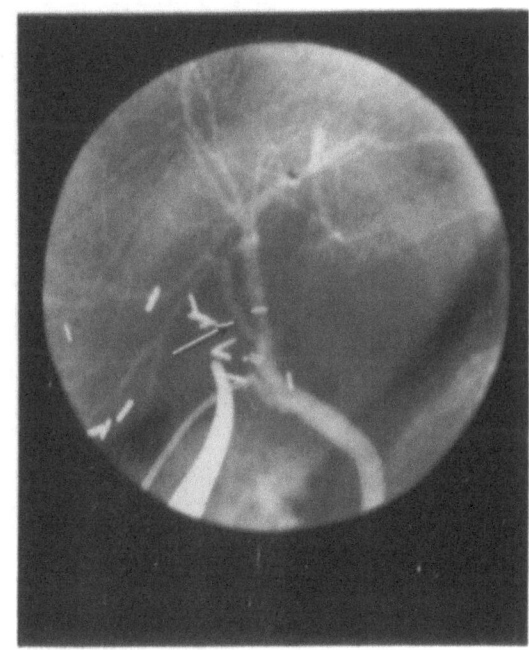

Fig. 4.12. Aberrant duct draining immediately above the cystic duct (arrow). Overlooking this anomaly could result in a biliary fistula or ligature of an important structure.

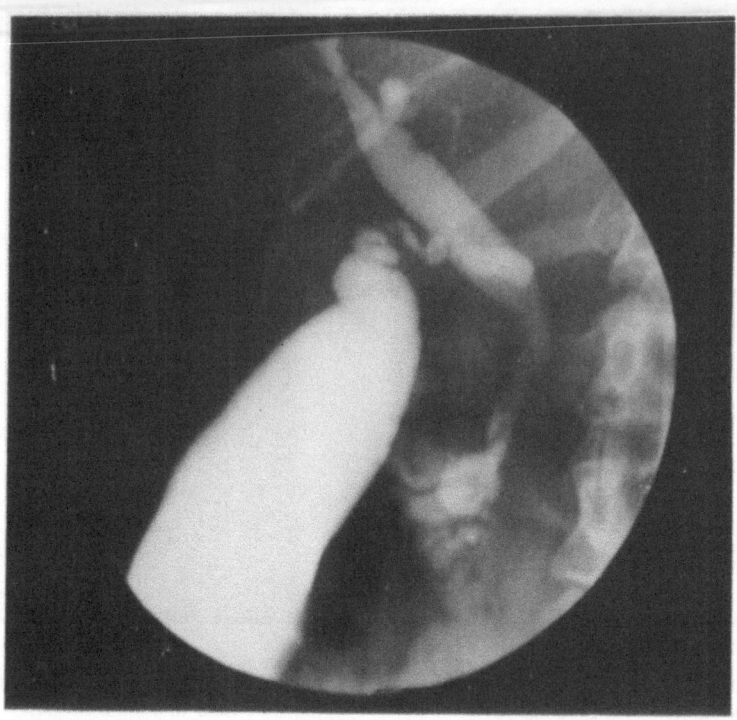

Fig. 4.13a. Cholecysto-cholangiogram. Note the choledochocele of the distal duct. These cases have a greater incidence of choledocholithiasis.

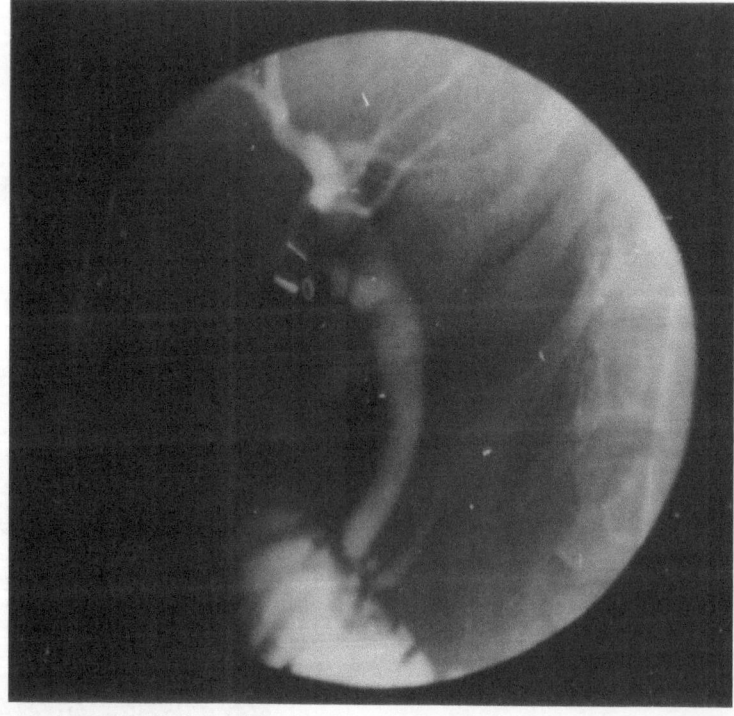

Fig. 4.13b. Small diverticulum of the distal duct. Pancreatic duct seen.

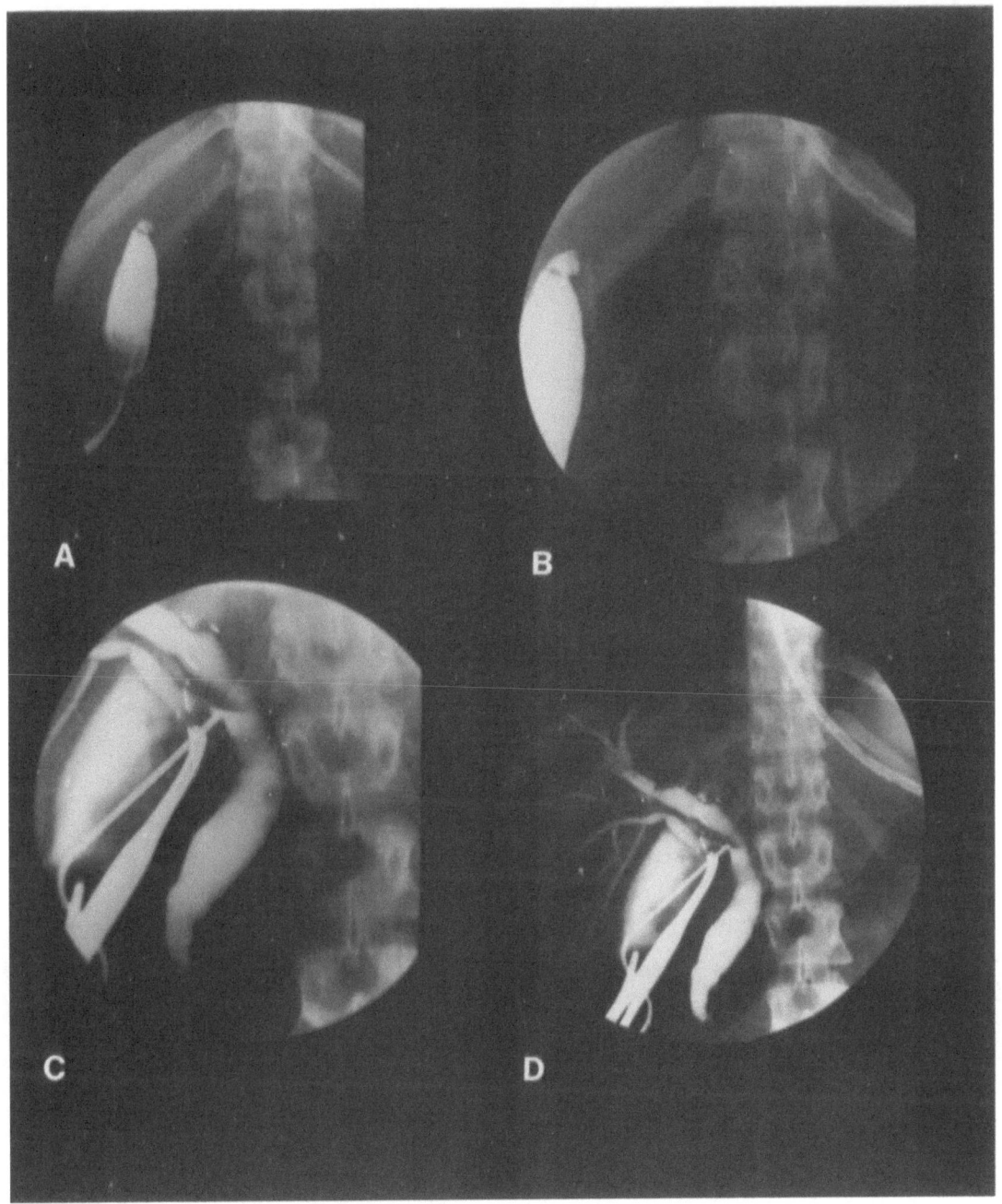

Figs. 4.14a–b. Cholecysto-cholangiogram demonstrates gallbladder neck obstruction and no information about the ductal system.
Figs. 4.14c–d. Ductal anatomy displayed in the same case after a cystic duct cholangiogram. The cystic duct joins the right hepatic duct.

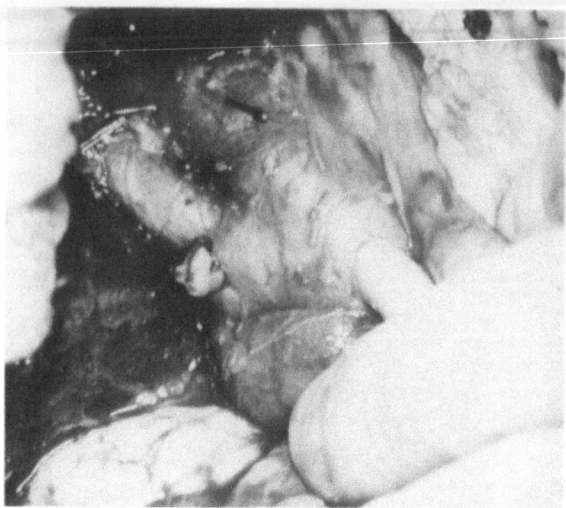

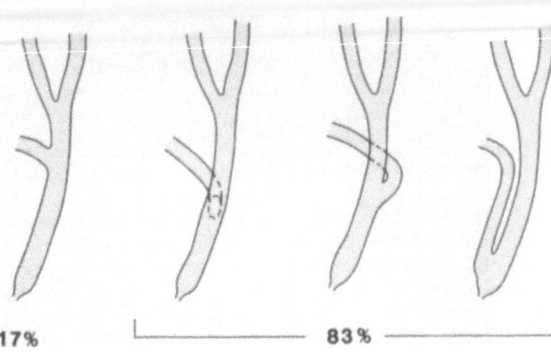

Fig. 4.14e. Black and white print of a color operative photograph showing, the short cystic duct ligated at the right hepatic branch. An iatrogenic injury was avoided by a timely display of the anatomy and important anomaly in this emergency case.

Fig. 4.15. Schematic diagram of cystic duct drainage into the common duct. In our material (1400 cholangiograms) only 17% entered the CBD from the lateral side. In 41% the duct joined anteriorly or posteriorly. In 35% the cystic duct spiraled posteriorly around the CBD to enter the medial aspect. Seven percent presented with parallel drainage. This indicates that in 83% a longer than expected cystic duct stump remains.

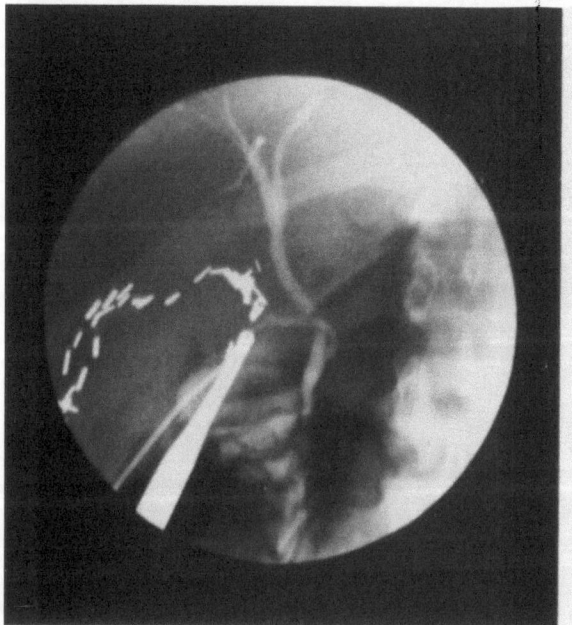

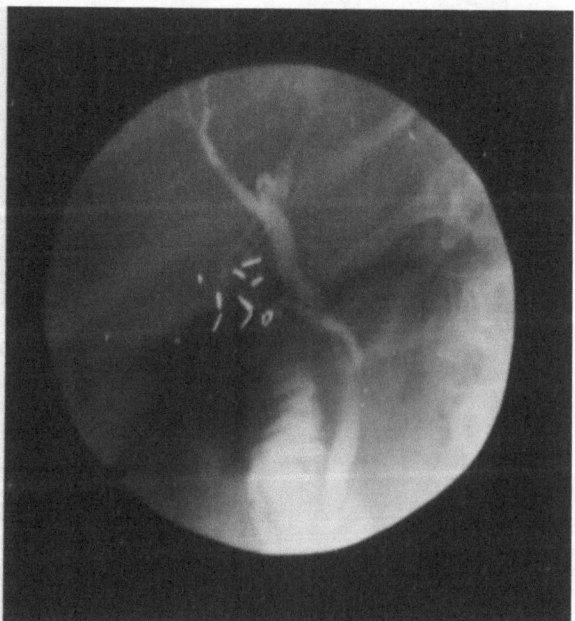

Fig. 4.16a–b. Typical examples of a spiral drainage of the cystic duct into the common bile duct.

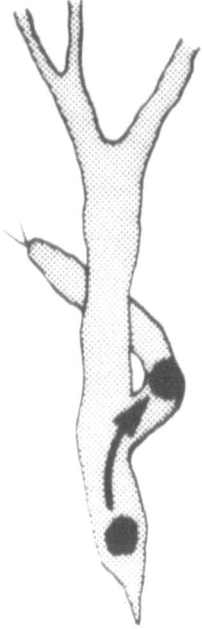

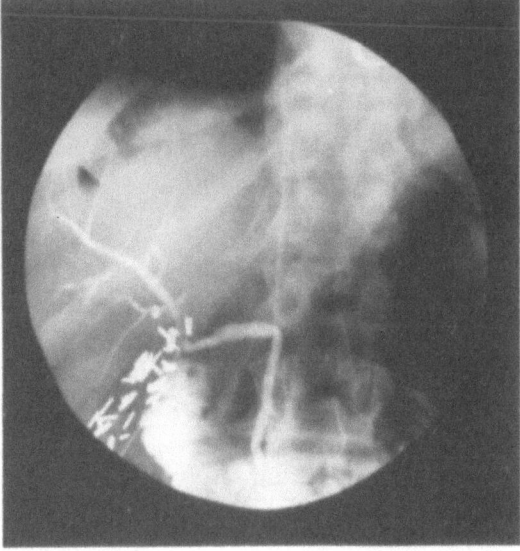

Fig. 4.17. In cases with choledocholithiasis and a dilated ductal system, a stone may be displaced into the enlarged cystic duct during the exploration and stone extraction procedure and not discovered until the postoperative T-tube cholangiogram (See Chapter 5 Operative Biliary Endoscopy).

Fig. 4.18. Low entry of the distal duct into the third portion of duodenum is not uncommon (For details see text Chapter 5 Operative Biliary Endoscopy).

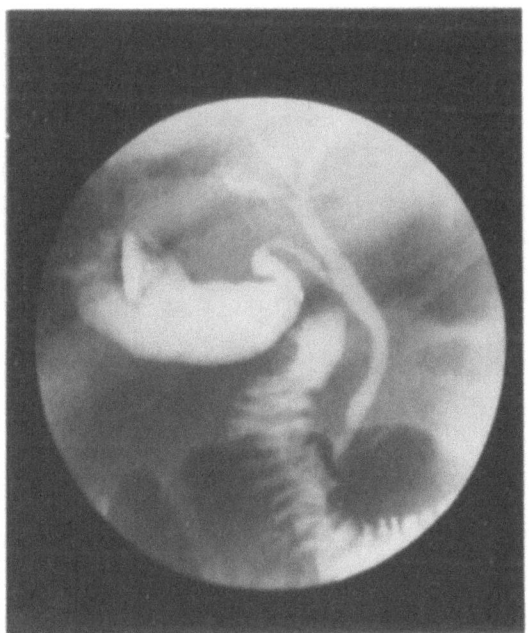

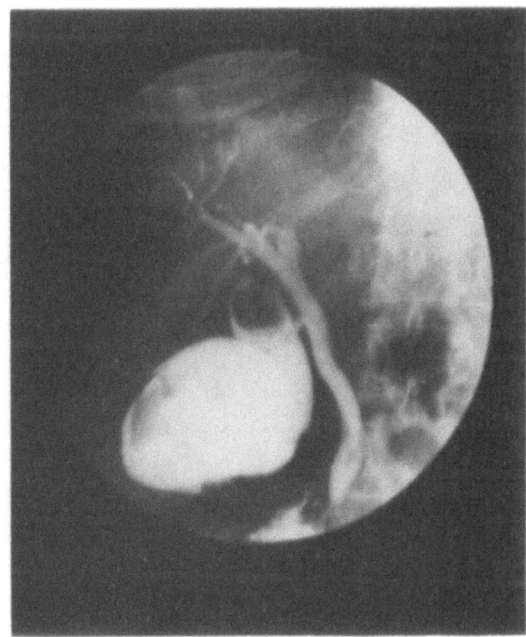

Fig. 4.19a. Cholecysto-cholangiogram displaying cholelithiasis, acute cholecystitis in a very ill patient with multiple organ failure. Cholecystotomy with removal of calculi was performed. As the cholangiogram revealed a normal appearing extra-hepatic biliary system, without stones, only a cholecystostomy was performed.

Fig. 4.19b. Cholecysto-Cholangiogram in another acute case. Note the large calculus in Hartmann's pouch almost impinging on the common hepatic duct. (Early stage of a Mirizzi's syndrome??) Spiral cystic duct with low drainage into common duct.

46

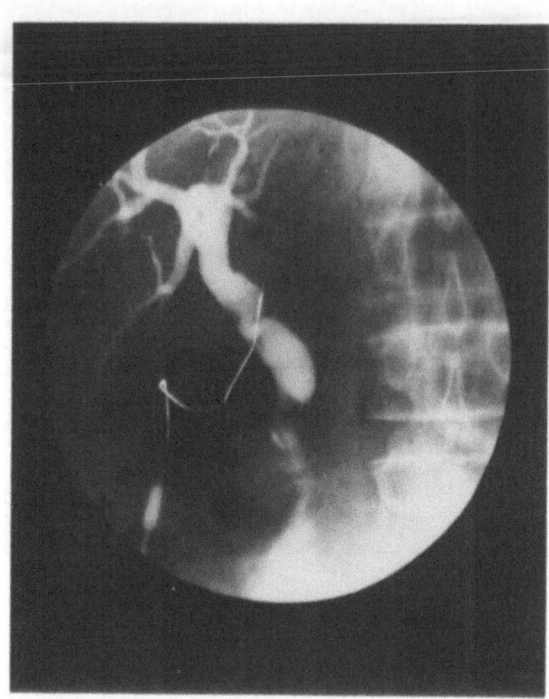

Fig. 4.20. Choledocho-cholangiogram during a secondary exploration. A butterfly needle with an extension tube is employed in this case. During the injection, back pressure can dislodge this small needle and extravasation and an incomplete cholangiogram will be the end result. Transfixation of the needle through the anterior wall with a fine stitch can be done, but the needle holes may also be the source of (contrast material) leakage.

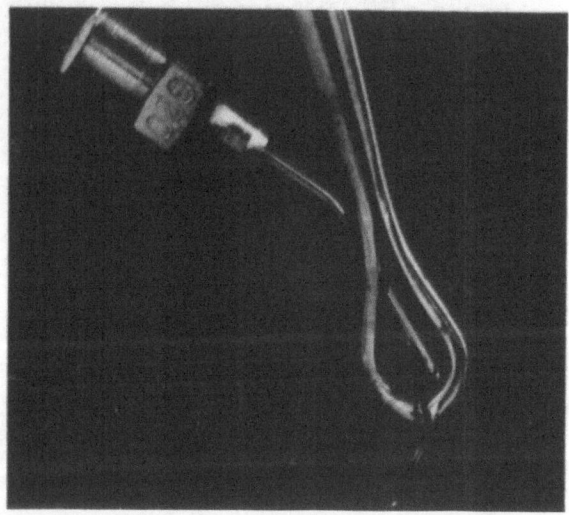

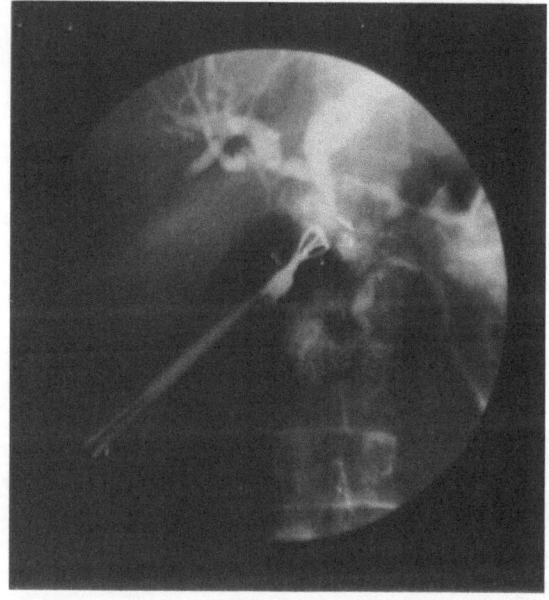

Fig. 4.21a. The Abbott needle. In one limb of a Babcock clamp a hole is drilled and a needle inserted and bent. The CBD is approached with this clamp in an open position. The anterior wall is penetrated. Through the connected venous extension tube, bile is aspirated and the clamp closed. The clamp encloses a part of the anterior wall fixing the needle in position.

Fig. 4.21b. The Abbott Clamp. This useful tool can be 'produced' in every hospital machine shop. Unless used with care, this clamps may cause damage to the ductal wall.

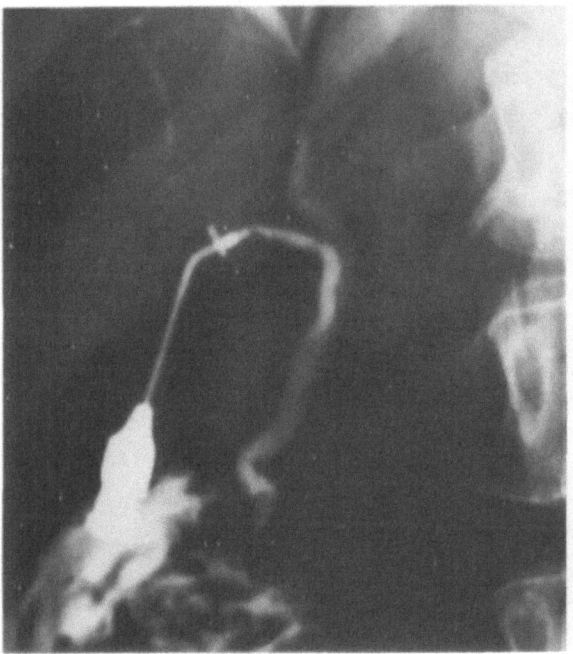

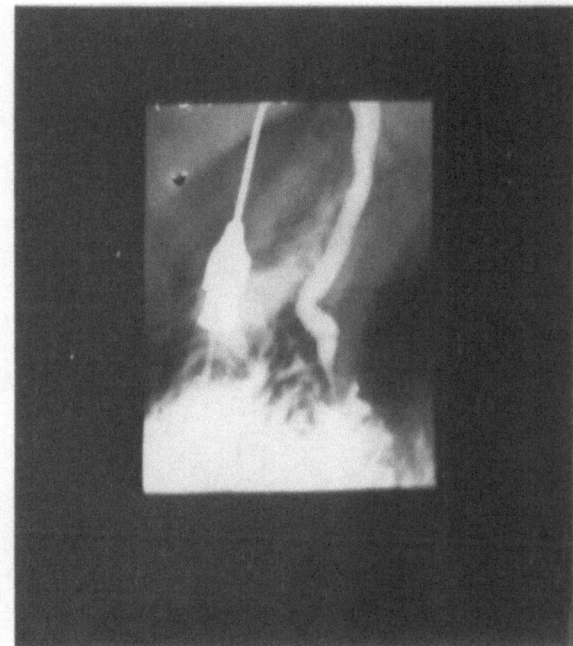

Fig. 4.22a. Operative transcystic standard cholangiogram demonstrating a normal ductal system with early filling at the duodenum, but insufficient detail of the peri-ampullary region.

Fig. 4.22b. Contact selective cholangiogram obtained in the same patient after insertion of a dental film in a sterile package behind the mobilized duodenum and head of pancreas. The film outlines the precise anatomy of the common channel with its mucosal folds in the inferior choledochal sphincter.

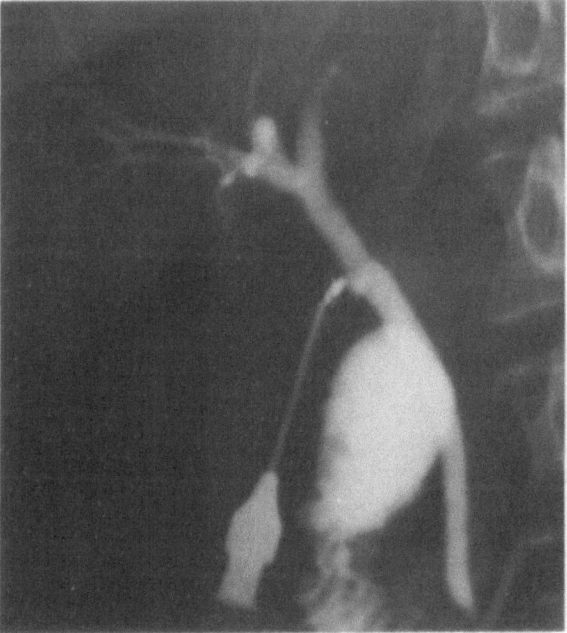

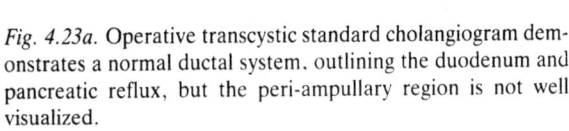

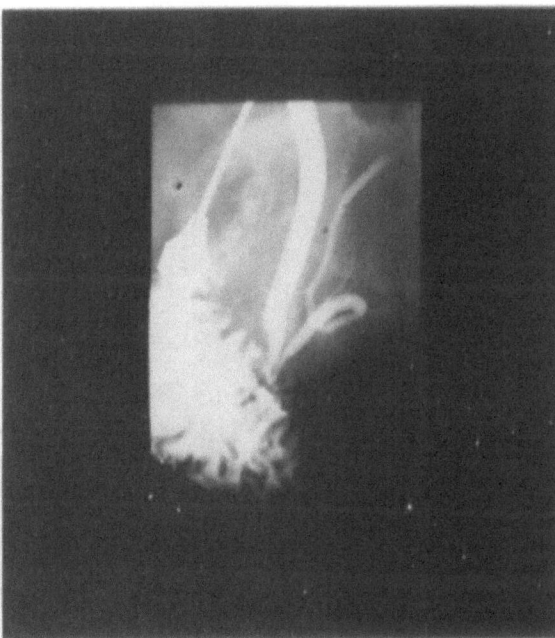

Fig. 4.23a. Operative transcystic standard cholangiogram demonstrates a normal ductal system, outlining the duodenum and pancreatic reflux, but the peri-ampullary region is not well visualized.

Fig. 4.23b. Contact selective cholangiogram in the same patient demonstrates clearly the peri-ampullary region. Both the choledochal and pancreatic sphincters are outlined. The anatomy of the pancreatic duct and its branches is also visualized.

48

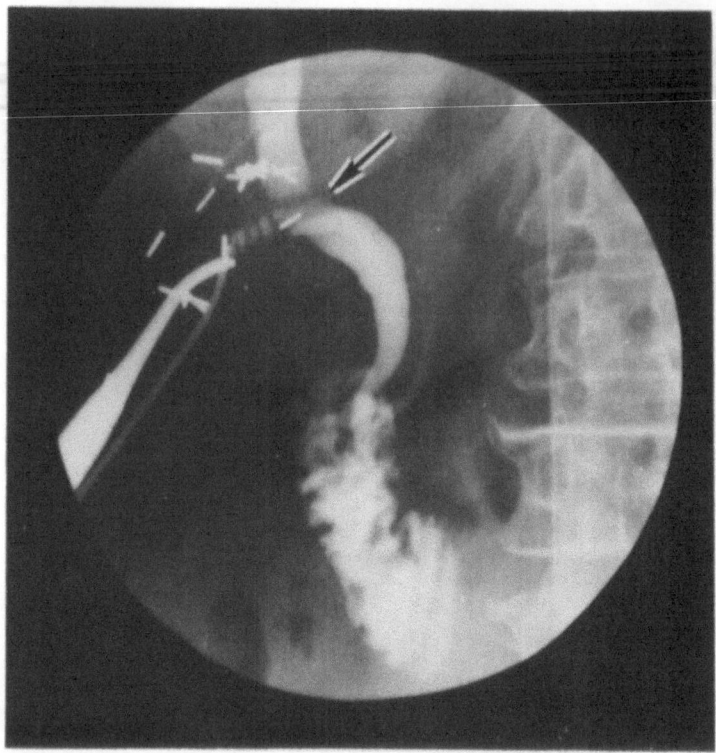

Fig. 4.24. A thin transverse radiolucency (arrow) crossing the common hepatic duct is due to a vascular impression (cystic duct artery or hepatic arterial branch).

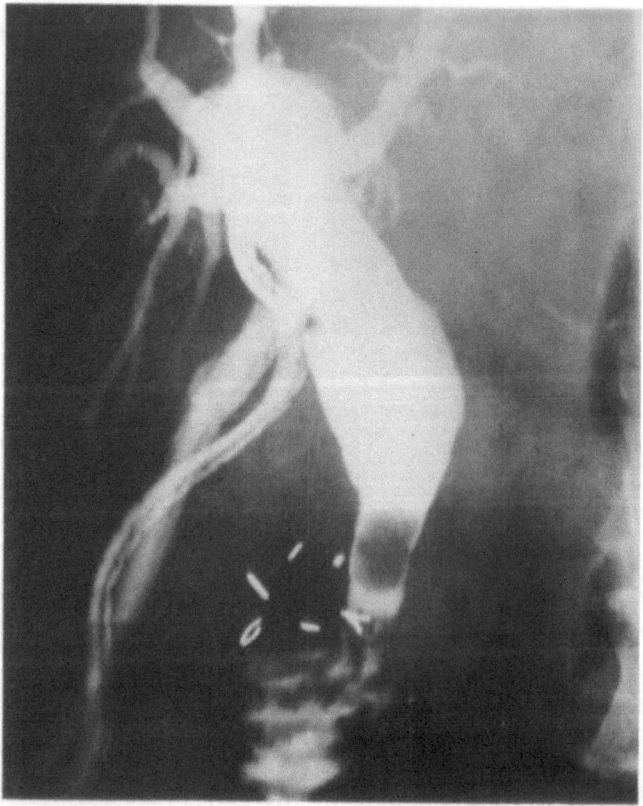

Fig. 4.25. In this patient a large ovoid filling defect was found on the postoperative T-tube cholangiogram and was referred to us for stone extraction through the T-tube tract. This 'calculus' proved to be a blood clot.

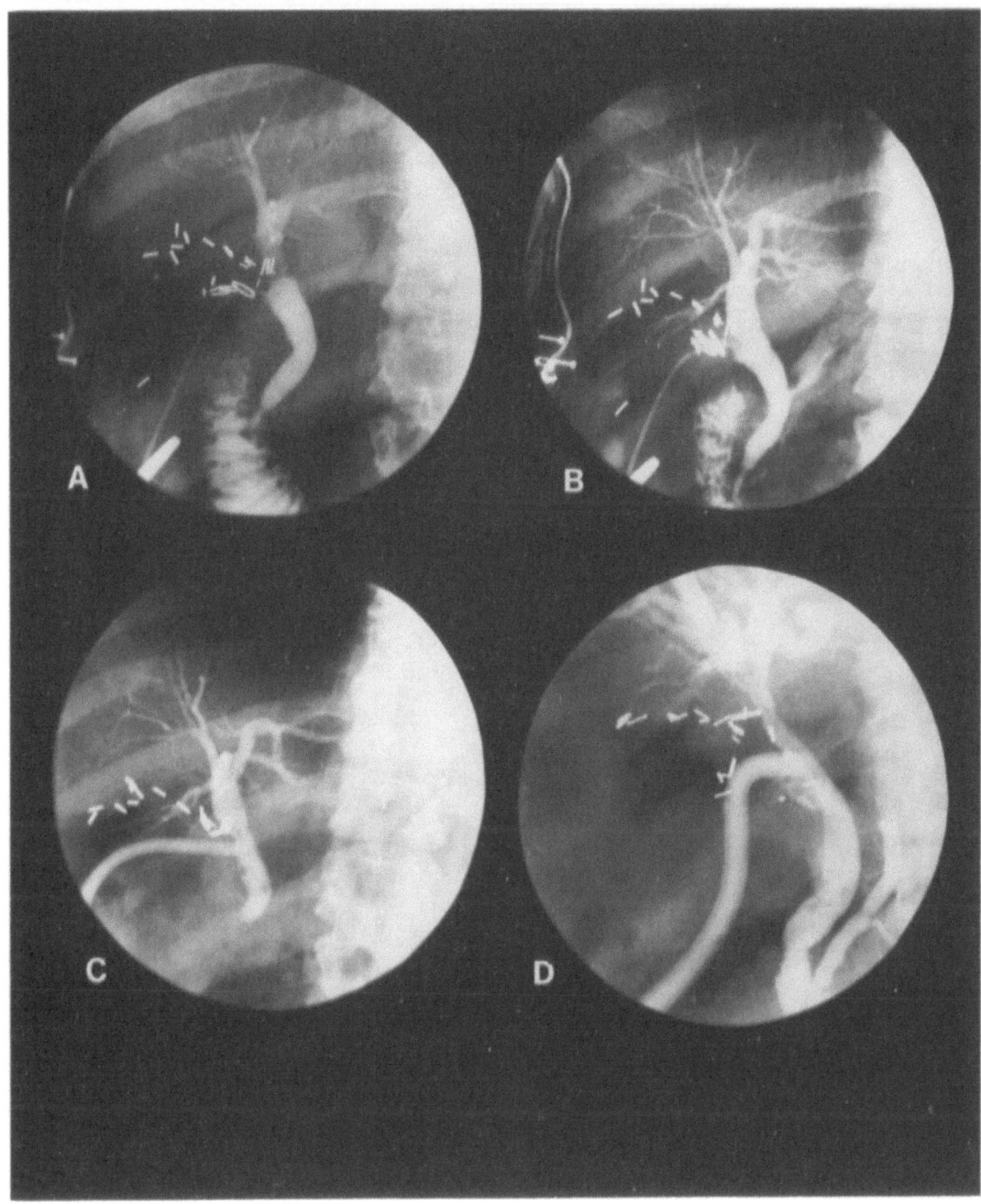

Figs. 4.26a–b. Cystic duct cholangiogram (two of eight films), interpreted as negative with no calculi, good sphincter function, and duodenal drainage. Because of the history (chills, jaundice, elevated liver function tests), the surgeon opened the duct and found cholangitis but no stones. Findings were supported by cholangioscopy.

Fig. 4.26c. Completion T-tube cholangiogram after manipulations. Note the number of small irregular lucencies produced by the desquamation of debris during duct exploration.

Fig. 4.26d. Completion cholangiogram of a different patient. Here stones were removed, but due to repeated instrumental manipulations, again lucencies were created by debris which is always present in cholangitis. One of the reasons why we recommend an initial radiological examination prior to choledochotomy is because it is performed in a closed system before the introduction of artifacts of manipulation.

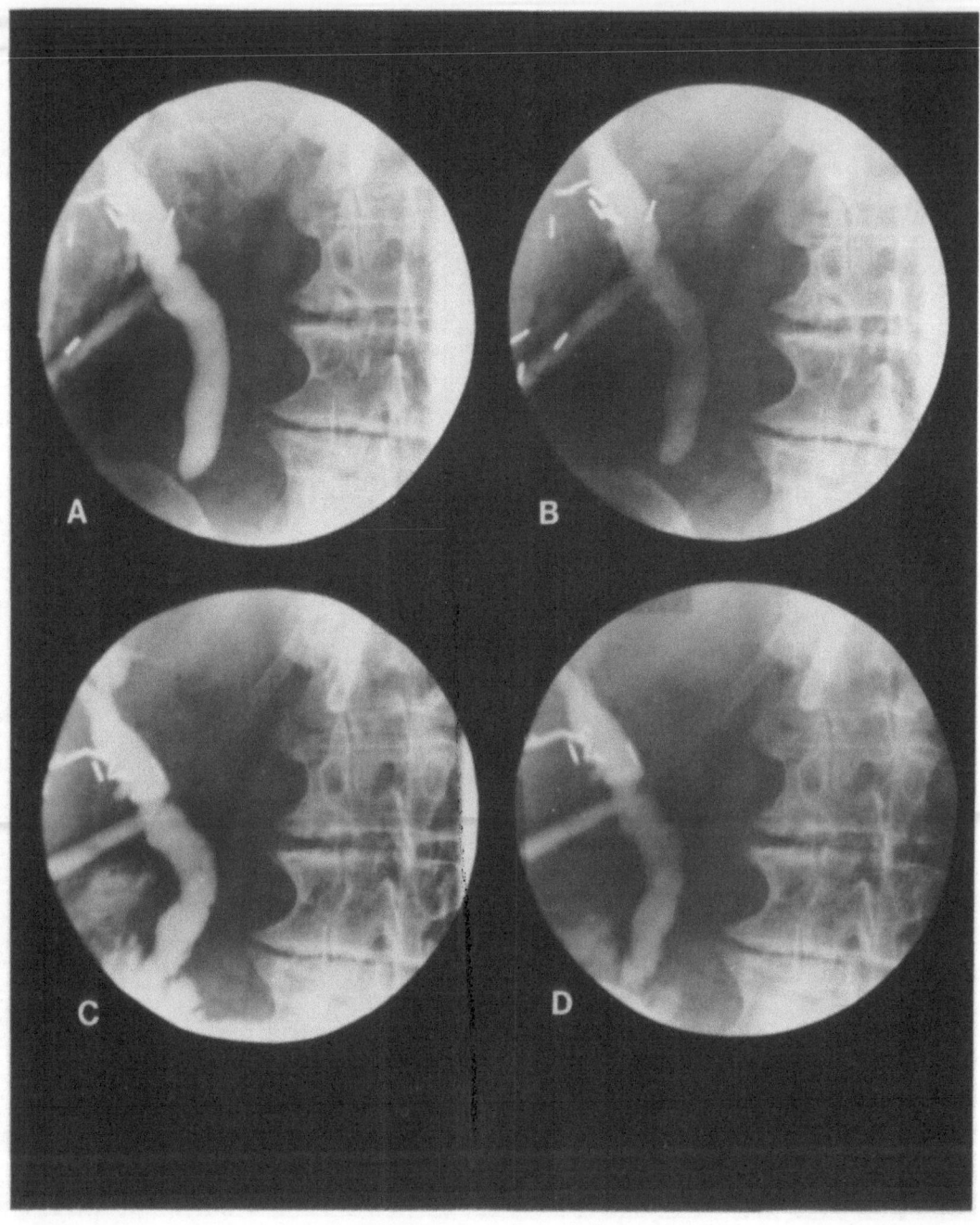

Figs. 4.27a–d. Sphincter spasm after manipulations. No contrast material enters the duodenum, a very common and sometimes frustrating phenomenon. If only one or two films are available (e.g. a and b), it would be difficult to differentiate spasm from an obstructing stone. When more exposures are available (c and d), calculus can be excluded with certainty and valuable operating time saved.

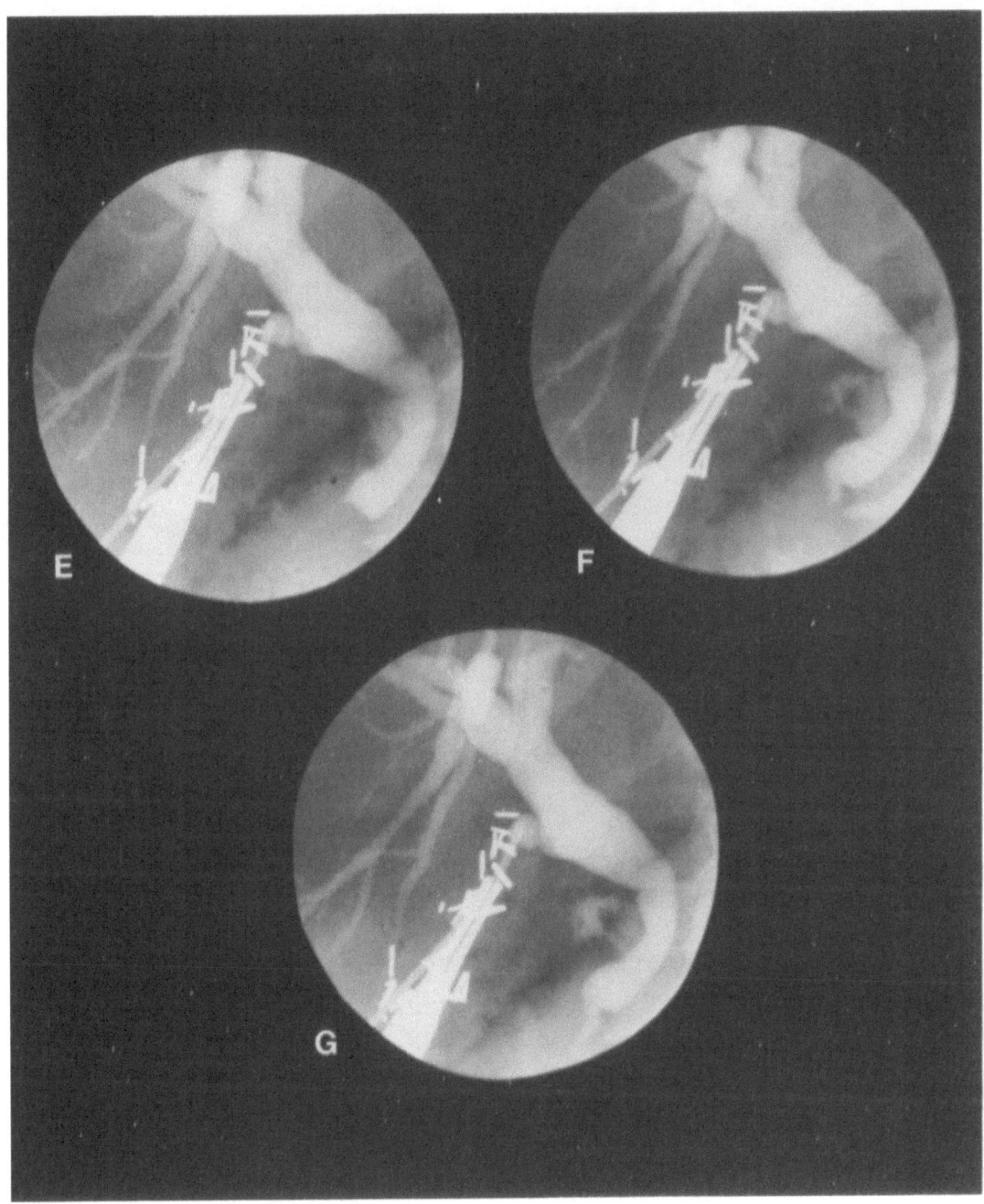

Figs. 4.27e–g. Same sphincter problem as mentioned under Figures 4.27a–d, but now with a characteristic thumbprint or 'pseudocalculus' sign (e). Films f and g (selected out of a series of eight) clearly demonstrate the entire cycle of sphincter function. Note dilated pancreatic duct (f).

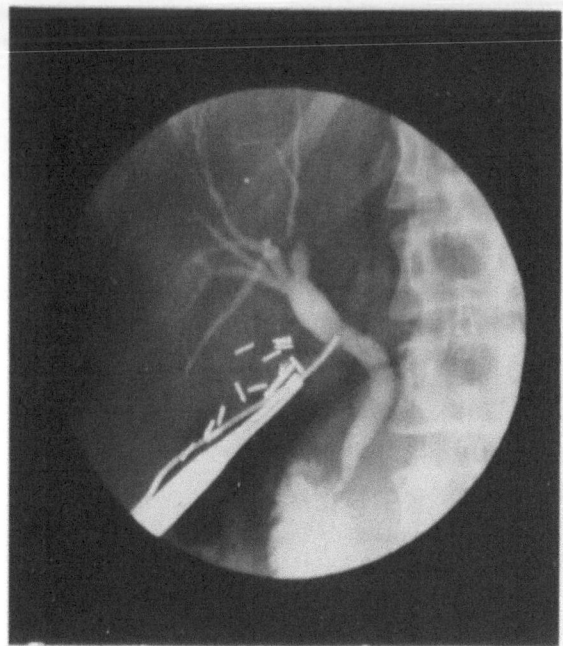

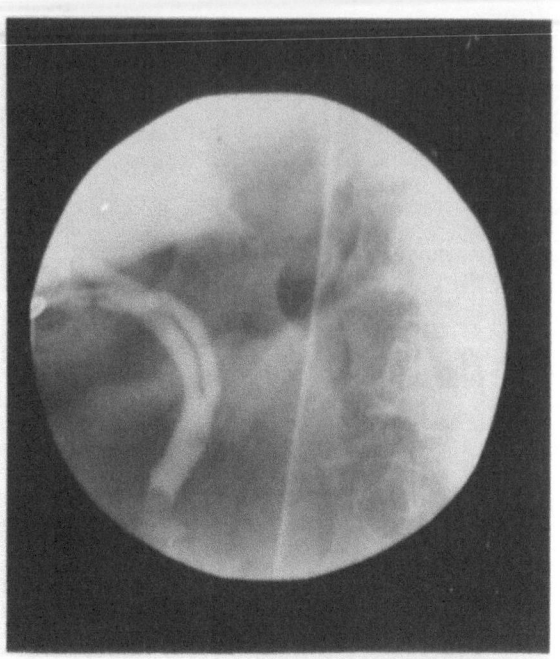

Fig. 4.28. In those few cases where an iodine hypersensitivity is present a suspension of sterile barium can be injected without any risk and a good contrast cholangiogram achieved (for details see text).

Fig. 4.29a. Cystic duct cholangiogram showing a spiral cystic duct and stones within the distal CBD.

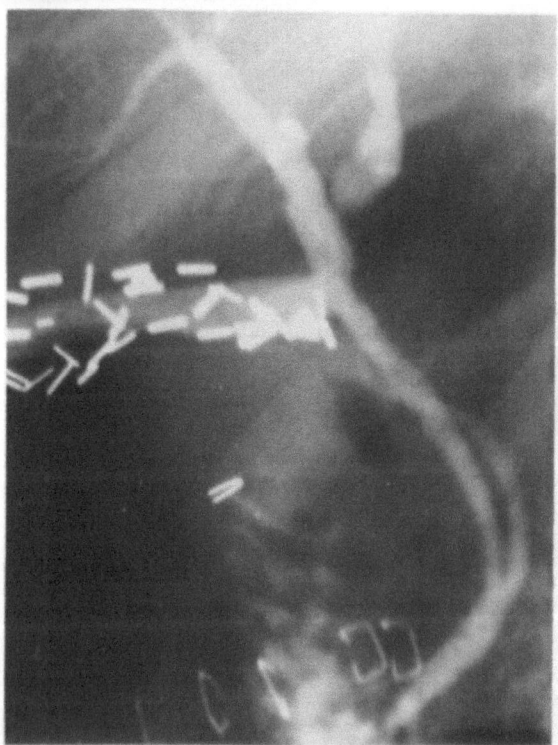

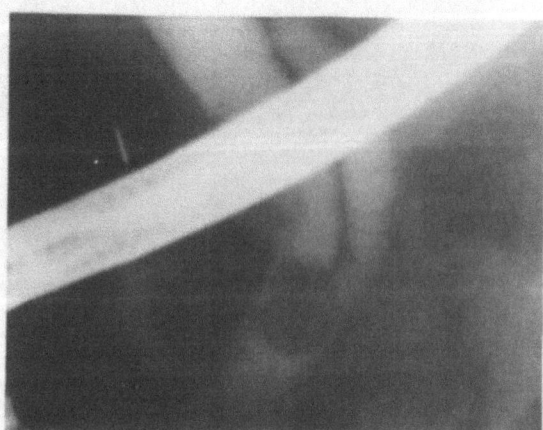

Fig. 4.29b. Postoperative T-tube cholangiogram displays a normal size CBD without calculi and with good duodenal drainage.

Fig. 4.29c. Retrograde cholangiogram two years later. Dilated ducts with stones in CBD.

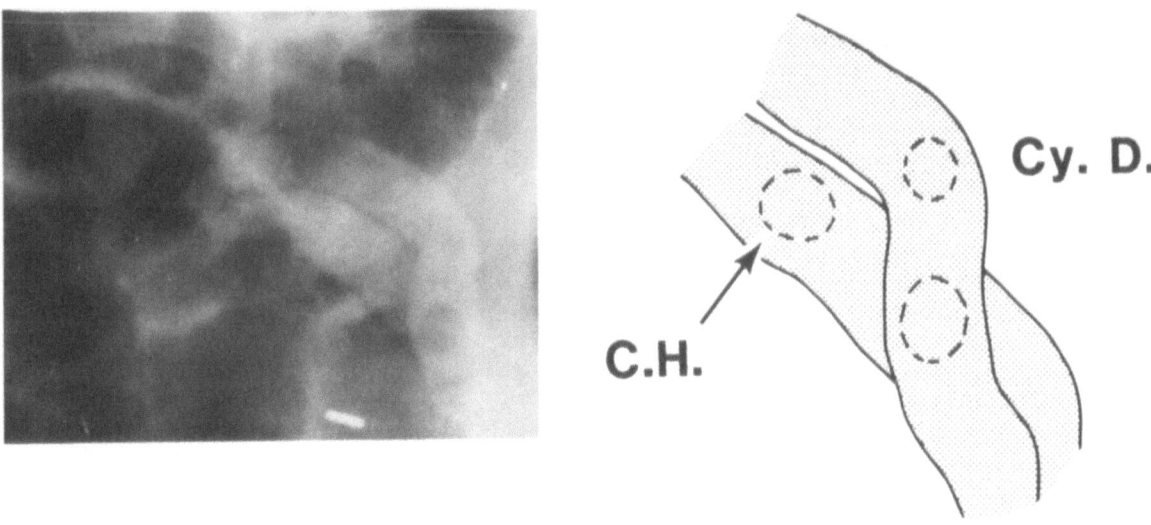

Fig. 4.29d. Retrograde cholangiogram; calculi in dilated spiral cystic duct remnant (diagram).

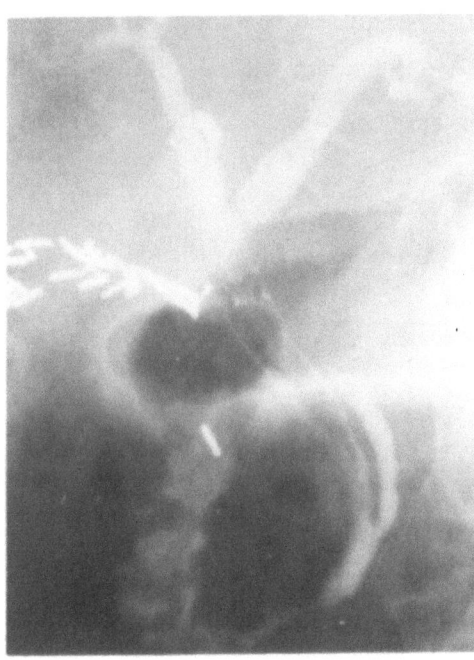

Fig. 4.29e. Retrograde cholangiogram post-endoscopic papillo-tomy; contrast material and gas in CBD. Diminished caliber of the ducts with passage of the calculi.

CHAPTER 5

OPERATIVE BILIARY ENDOSCOPY (CHOLANGIOSCOPY)

1. Introduction

Despite the frequency of choledochotomy the bile duct was virtually the last hollow viscus for which endoscopy was developed. The enthusiasm for operative cholangioscopy and limitations of the early endoscopes probably account for this delay (1–8). The biliary tract, unlike other organs, presents a special challenge for the endoscopist. The technique must be carried out under strict sterile conditions. These requirements perhaps inhibited successful application until the recent revolution in optical technology. Initial expectations of flexible fiber optics were thwarted because of the complexity related to manipulation difficulties with repeated sterilization of these expensive instruments, and the inferior image quality (9–10). At the present stage of optical technology a modern rigid system provides a better image that the flexible fiberoptic one. The rigid scope is much simpler to manipulate and easier to learn (11).

The rapid world-wide acceptance of cholangioscopy of the common bile duct (CBD) indicated the importance of this valuable adjunct. Following the early enthusiasts, the incidence of missed stones decreased (1–3%) (12–16), but subsequent publications indicated that the results did not reduce missed stone rate significantly (4–9%) (17–18).

We thought that it would be important to draw attention to certain steps of intraoperative preparation and technique which is the key to biliary endoscopy, resulting in more acceptable results without jeopardizing the effectiveness of the procedure.

Regarding terminology, we prefer the term 'cholangioscopy' rather than 'choledochoscopy' because the intraparenchymal ductal system is also inspected in addition to the choledochus.

2. Instrumentation

The rigid cholangioscope consists of a right angled telescope with a built-in irrigation channel with a fiberoptic light carrier. The outside diameter is 5×3 mm and allows its insertion even into a nondilated duct. The standard 40 mm horizontal limb usually suffices, but on occasion the distal duct can be long and the 60 mm scope is needed to visualize the ampulla (Figs. 5.1a–c). *It is of utmost importance to obtain an initial cholangiogram to see the drainage site and configuration of the distal duct,* because this will determine which scope should be employed (the shorter or the longer one) and what type of difficulties can be anticipated because of the long or tortuous drainage into the duodenum (Fig. 5.2) (19, 20).

2.1. Accessories

The attachable instrument channel is one of the most important accessories (Fig. 5.3). In case of choledocholithiasis it *should be immediately introduced with the scope* and instead of blind manipulations, the Dormia stone basket applied (Fig. 5.4). Calculi should be entrapped accurately with precision, under visual control. The same instrument channel can be employed for the use of a Fr. 4 balloon catheter (Fig. 5.5). In case of manipulations (Dormia basket) an assistant is required, and therefore a teaching attachment is coupled to the endoscope. This provides the possibility of simultaneous observation and coordination of extraction maneuvers (Fig. 5.2–1).

Before the era of biliary endoscopy the biliary (balloon) catheter was introduced blindly into the duodenum, inflated and palpated. During withdrawal we have to deflate the balloon to be able to pass the sphincter. During this maneuver the *balloon suddenly jumps* and dispite immediate reinflation, a calculus, located near the ampulla or sphincter, can be bypassed.

The same maneuver can be now performed *under endoscopic control,* advancing the balloon catheter into the duodenum through the instrument channel and withdrawing it partially desufflated and reinflating it but this time seeing the position clearly in relation to the sphincter and calculus. Impacted stones can be removed with the Dormia basket, balloon catheter or an attachable stone forceps (Figs. 5.2g and 5.6). In general the Dormia basket and balloon catheter are the major tools for stone extractions.

To provide adequate irrigation for proper distention and clearing of the ducts, the Fenwal pressure irrigation system is employed (Fig. 5.7). A cuff pressure of 150–200 mm/Hg monitored by a manometer, ensures optimal visualization. The saline fluid is delivered to the bile ducts under low pressure because of the high resistance of the narrow irrigation channel. A saline drip under hydrostatic pressure only will not suffice the conditions. Optimally, illumination is provided from an external light source via a flexible fiberoptic cable (Fig. 5.2k). An attachable biopsy forceps is provided to obtain tissue samples of suspicious areas (Fig. 5.8).

3. Technique

A small (10 mm) standard choledochotomy incision is suitable for the introduction of the scope. The incision should not be too long, to avoid excessive leakage of the irrigation fluid, and a suction tube should be placed beside the CBD to remove the overflow (Fig. 5.9). The introduction of the scope is aided by stay sutures which open the lumen. Stay sutures inserted into the CBD wall and held by hemostats can be crossed after the introduction of the scope, decreasing leakage (Fig. 5.10).

3.1. Mobilization of the duodenum
The most important step which is overlooked and is probably the factor in the majority of cases of unsuccessful endoscopic procedures of the (distal) biliary system, or missed stones, is the omission or insufficient mobilization of the duodenum. It is not enough to divide the peritoneal reflection of the anti-mesenteric border of the second part of the duodenum, but it is also important to mobilize with sharp and blunt dissection the duodenum. Sometimes the superior mesenteric vein will come into vision. Only if the duodenum is widely mobilized can it be kept on a proper stretch to straighten a tortuous or curved distal duct to facilitate proper visualization. During the endoscopic examination, one hand must always be placed on the mobilized duodenum whereby the introduced cholangioscope can be felt as a probe and the wall of the duct in front of the scope is stretched and kept straight to provide optimal vision by applying continuous traction. It is not necessary to introduce the scope through the sphincter into the duodenum if the sphincter is well observed (Figs. 5.11, 5.12, 5.13, 5.14, 5.15).

The attachment of a disc to the eyepiece can protect it from touching the face mask (Fig. 5.2d). It is very important that before the procedure is started, the operator should check with the scrub nurse that the scope and its accessories are available and the entire set is in operational condition. It is advisable to keep the cholangioscope on a separate (sterile) table and not to mix it with other surgical hand instruments.

3.2 Endoscopic appearance
When the scope is first introduced a yellowish or red circle will be seen only. This indicates that the objective or working tip is in contact with the ductal wall. It can be corrected by a slow withdrawal or tilting of the scope slightly until, in case of the distal duct, the sphincter is seen, or, in case of the proximal insertion, the bifurcation. The best views are generally obtained during withdrawal of the scope followed by slow readvancement, but this time under visual control (Figs. 5.16a–d and 5.17a–b).

After satisfactory endoscopy of the distal duct, the scope is withdrawn, rotated 180° and reintroduced towards the hepatic ducts (Figs. 5.18a–b and 5.19a–b). Once the bifurcation is identified the scope is rotated to bring the right main orifice into view. It is then advanced along the tributary as far as possible. There is a large variation of normal anatomy, but after a few cases, one accumulates enough experience to examine each orifice systematically. Upon slow withdrawal of the scope the bifurcation turns into view. Slight rotation to the right reveals the orifice of the left main duct which is then followed peripherally. It is not unusual to be able to see even tertiary bifurcations.

3.3 The cystic stump remnant

In 83% a long, parallel, or spiral course of the dilated duct is present (19). This will result in a long cystic stump remnant. A small calculus, after prolonged manipulations, can disappear in this hidden space with ease. We should remember this possibility in cases with dilated ducts and multiple stones, and before completing the procedure, it is advisable to introduce a flexible probe or catheter through the dilated cystic duct stump into the CBD. This will deliver any calculi from this 'blind pouch' into the main duct. On repeat endoscopy these calculi can be detected and removed. This step will prevent the not uncommon incidence of a retained cystic duct stone migrating into the CBD at a later stage (See Chapter 4 Operative Cholangiography: Figs. 4.15, 4.17 and 4.18).

4. Endoscopic anatomy and pathology

4.1 Normal findings

The mucous membrane of the CBD has a pale, pinkish, yellowish appearance. There are some longitudinal folds, which are flattened by the pressure of the irrigating fluid. Delicate submucosal vascular reticulum is usually visible. Approaching the ampulla our path will become narrower, funnel-shaped and curved towards the right posteriorly. The sphincter area, itself, has a characteristic appearance which must be identified to ensure complete distal examination. The orifice is outlined against the dark background of the adjacent duodenal lumen. It appears usually 'stellate' but may look like a 'fishmouth,' 'pinpoint,' or 'patulous' opening. The mucosa, at this point, is coarser and is raised into folds, covered sometimes by fibrinous exudate. Failure to visualize this structure precludes any diagnostic conclusions regarding the state of the distal duct. The orifice of the pancreatic duct is rarely visualized (Figs. 5.20a–d). The bifurcation of the common hepatic duct is similar in appearance to the bronchial carina. The right hepatic duct divides shortly into the two segmental divisions, whereas the left duct usually has no major visible tributaries. The mucosa of the hepatic duct is paler than that of the distal duct. Variations in the hepatic ductal anatomy or orifices are very common (20). The segmental divisions of the right hepatic duct may join the left hepatic duct at the same level, giving the appearance of a trifurcation. The ducts may be dilated, allowing the examination of the tertiary (subsegmental) hepatic ducts. The identification of the major bifurcation is mandatory to achieve hepatic duct visualization (Fig. 5.21a–d).

4.2 Cholangitis

It is a very common finding in patients with choledocholithiasis and can be of varying degree, ranging from a mucosal congestion and edema to marked ulcerative cholangitis with fibrinous exudate. These inflammatory changes become more marked towards the ampulla. At times the examination of the sphincter area is obscured by an inflammatory exudate which accumulates in this region. Removal of these debris by irrigation or Randall stone forceps, after temporary withdrawal of the scope is usually rewarded by vastly improved visualization. Changes are far less conspicuous in the hepatic ducts.

4.3 Calculi

Stones are easily identified endoscopically and may be free-floating or rolling around from the irrigation fluid and can be sometimes evacuated spontaneously on withdrawal of the instrument due to the irrigating stream. At times a stone can be found impacted in the orifice of the hepatic duct or ampulla, partially embedded in the duct wall or in a diverticulum of the distal duct. Multiple stones and biliary mud are frequently found behind a large calculus. Repeat endoscopic examination is necessary to ensure complete stone-free ducts. In case of hepatic stones it is important to manipulate with precision (e.g. to move carefully the basket or balloon beyond the calculus) to avoid bleeding, impaction or further advancement into the periphery (Figs. 5.22a–c and 5.23a–c).

4.4 Ampullary stenosis

The normal looking ampulla appears to be soft and pliable and often can be seen during the opening and closing phase by pressure of the irrigating

58

Table 5.1.[a]

	Year	Retained stones per cholangio scopies	Per cent retained stones
Wildegans (2)	1958	1/165	0.6
Berci (4)	1961	1/12	8.3
Leslie (12)	1962	1/37	2.7
Schein (6)	1962	1/117	0.9
Shore (7)	1962	2/100	2.0
Longland (22)	1973	6/37	16.0
Ottinger, Warshaw *et al.* (23)	1974	1/22	4.5
Griffin (24)	1976	0/32	0.0
Nora, Berci *et al.* (15)	1976	9/215	2.7
Shore and Berci (11)	1976	3/120	2.5
Finnis and Rowntree (25)	1977	0/88	0.0
Ashby (26)	1978	0/46	0.0
Fortanier, Lacroix *et al.* (27)	1978	1/99	1.0
Kappas, A. Williams *et al.* (28)	1979	12/121	10.0
Botticher and Knoch (29)	1980	1/76	1.3
Feliciano, Mattox, *et al.* (17)	1980	7/140	8.9
Lennert (30)	1980	1/150	1.1
Yap, Atacador *et al.* (31)	1980	4/149	2.7
Motson, Wood *et al.* (32)	1980	2/50	4.0
Bauer, Salky *et al.* (33)	1981	1/50	2.0
Rattner and Warshaw (18)	1981	6/144	4.1
Reitsma (13)	1981	3/137	2.9
Kappes, Wilson *et al.* (34)	1982	3/148	2.0
IBA (35)	1982	8/182	4.4
CSMC (36)	1983	4/108	3.7
Cuschieri (pers. comm.)	1983	3/127	2.4

[a] The above collected data from the literature show a great variation in the incidence of missed stones (0 to 16%). It could be that the first 30 or 40 procedures were flawless and during the next five cases one or two stones were overlooked. Therefore, a larger series is required to obtain a more realistic picture.

There are certain criteria which have to be fulfilled (for details see text) to enable us to compare these results in a more realistic, objective way. The percentage of negative explorations in some of the above quoted papers was surprisingly high (10 to 20%).

stream. Stenosis of the sphincter presents as a pinpoint opening beyond a distended common duct simulating the entrance to a 'tunnel.' The appearance is not diagnostic, however, because it can be caused by a spasm of the sphincter of Oddi, frequently encountered after manipulations.

4.5 Neoplasms

Papillary tumors protruding through the biliary lumen are well seen. They can be biopsied with the forceps described amongst the accessories. Partial or complete extrinsic ductal obstruction due to a carcinoma of the extra-ductal origin (pancreas, metastases, periductal lymph nodes, lymphoma, etc.) can be encountered. Endoscopic appearance is usually one of the sudden complete occlusion of the ductal lumen through which the scope cannot be advanced. The tumor itself, is rarely visualized, nor can it be biopsied. Extrinsic compression of the distal CBD by an inflammatory mass in the head of the pancreas is indistinguishable from a malignant lesion.

4.6 Miscellaneous

Benign tumors of the CBD, diverticulum of the distal duct, congenital webs, foreign bodies, and parasites are rare.

5. Repeat cholangioscopy

It is advisable to keep the entire endoscopic set on a separate sterile instrument table in case of repeat use. In patients with difficult anatomy, inflammed edematous ducts or severe cholangitis, it is sometimes necessary to reintroduce the scope just to make sure that the stones are completely removed. In questionable completion cholangiograms, where debris can simulate a calculus, the repeat endoscopic procedure can produce the right answer. In choledocholithiasis with dilated ducts and dilated cystic stump, after completion of manipulations or scooping, it is advisable to reopen the ligated stump and pass a catheter or probe gently into the CBD and rescope the patient just to make sure that during the maneuvers a calculus has not moved and lies hidden in the cystic duct (under c. Cystic Stump). When the duct is re-endoscoped this stone can be discovered. Cases of multiple calculi, biliary mud or large number of smaller calculi in the periphery of hepatic ducts can give the impression of a technically intractable situation, and therefore, rescoping helps in decision making (bilio-enteric bypass).

6. Complications

Both authors (G.B. and A.C.) followed over 500 cholangioscopies and are not aware of any perforation of the distal CBD or major complication (bleeding, hemobilia) from the hepatic ducts after this endoscopic procedure.

The incidence of wound infection was not increased in cases where the endoscope was employed intraoperatively.

7. General aspects

7.1. Sterilization
We prefer gas sterilization. With our system the entire set with all accessories are wrapped and kept in one case. This is much easier for the nurses and ensures against loss or misplacement of instruments and accessories. We have two sets; therefore, two consecutive cases can be done per day if necessary. If only one set is available and there are two cases the same day, the telescopes and the basket can be soaked and rinsed, but the metal accessories (instrument channel) and biopsy or stone forceps can be flash autoclaved.

We do not recommend flash autoclaving of the telescope.

In case of flexible instruments, gas autoclaving is the method of choice.

7.2. Maintenance
This aspect is sometimes neglected or overlooked by surgeons. It is of paramount importance that a few nurses or O.R. technicians should be especially acquainted or trained in the cleaning, maintenance, assembly, and general knowledge of instrument functions. It could be a disaster if it is handled by a person who is not informed and does not know the important details of this process. We can end up with a very high repair and exchange cost of these delicate instruments. We have certain choledocho-

scopes which have been in use for six years without damage due to exquisite care by our nursing and technician staff, because we have taken the time to initiate a proper training program for endoscopic instruments.

8. Evaluation of results

We collected data from the literature (Table 5.1), and after careful scrutiny of the reports, we came to the conclusion that there is a definite necessity to establish certain criteria how results in this particular application of endoscopy should be collected and evaluated to enable us to compare them in a more realistic way.

(a) Those patients where primary closure of the CBD followed cholangioscopy should be excluded.

(b) Entero-biliary bypass cases should be analyzed separately.

(c) Cases where postoperative T-tube cholangiography is not available for one reason or the other, should be excluded from the evaluation.

(d) Intractable stones seen, but unable to be removed, should be listed separately.

(e) Primary cases should be differentiated from secondary explorations.

(f) The length or follow-up of patients should be recorded.

(g) The reported experience should be a minimum of 100 or more endoscoped cases.

9. Conclusions

Success in biliary endoscopy is *not only dependent* on the skill with the endoscopic procedure, but also on expeditious biliary surgery. The differences between the experienced and occasional cholangioscopist directly correlate with experience in CBD explorations (37).

We found modern operative cholangiography of utmost importance and help in obtaining additional information which is of value to the endoscopist (19, 20, 21).

It is apparent that in order to duplicate the best results it would be advisable to organize post-graduate teaching courses mainly with workshops where the technique can be taught on a one-to-one basis on biliary models or on experimental animals. The vena cava of an adult dog is a very good example where stone retrieval attempts can be practiced and experience accumulated with the various maneuvers.

The well motivated biliary surgeon can quickly become a master endoscopist if this important adjunct is taken seriously enough using the opportunity and procedures mentioned above.

The retained stone problem can be decreased significantly if biliary endoscopy is applied with appropriate know-how. It is also of equal importance to have accurate records and follow-up figures available from a longer time period (years). In our opinion this can be achieved only if one particular radiologist (who is interested in biliary cases) collects and *reviews every operative and postoperative T-tube cholangiogram* for over a minimum period of two to three years. If these X-ray films are reviewed by several members of a busy X-ray department, independently a missed stone may well not be included in the general evaluation or assessment. The results or interesting facets of biliary cases should be audited on an annual basis with detailed evaluation of the complications.

Regarding instrumentation, it does not make any difference which type of instrument is employed as long as the operator is familiar with it. The preparation of the duodenum and its generous mobilization is often omitted and is one of the main sources of technically inadequate examinations of the distal duct resulting in a retained stone.

In our experience and the experience of others the rigid type of cholangioscope is simpler to use and easier to learn for the general surgeon who is not an endoscopist (38).

It is encouraging that the American Board of Surgery included in its teaching program the necessity to learn surgical endoscopic procedures including operative biliary endoscopy which will show the positive results in a few years time.

The procedure itself is a great step forward since it allows intraoperative endoscopic removal of calculi without risk or increased morbidity. However it has to be clearly understood that purchasing the equipment is not enough. The operator has to be aware of the techniques in detail before applying it to man.

With routine cholangioscopy it should be possible to reduce the overall incidence of missed stone rate from the present level of 10–15% to 3%. This would constitute a significant advance.

In those few unfortunate cases where residual stones are observed on the postoperative T-tube cholangiogram, removal via the T-tube tract is possible in 90–95% of cases. The success of this procedure is enhanced if the T-tube is large and its tract relatively straight (Figs. 5.24a–d).

References

1. Bakes J: Die Choledochopapilloskopie. Arch Klin Chir 126:473–483, 1923.
2. Wildegans H: Grenzen der cholangiography und Aussicten der Endoskopie der tiefen Gallenwege. Med Klin 48:1270–1272, 1953.
3. Wildegans H: Die operative Gallengangsendoskopie. Munich, Urban & Schwartzenberg, 1960.
4. Berci G: Choledochoscopy. Med J Aust 2:861–863, 1961.
5. McIver MA: An instrument for visualizing the interior of the common duct at operation. Surgery 9:112–114, 1941.
6. Schein CJ: Biliary endoscopy: an appraisal of its value in biliary lithiasis. Surgery 65:1004–1008, 1969.
7. Shore JM, Lippman HN: Operative endoscopy of the biliary tract. Ann Surg 156:951–955, 1962.
8. Shore JM, Shore E: Operative biliary endoscopy. Ann Surg 171:269–277, 1970.
9. Shore JM, Lippman HN: A flexible choledochoscope. Lancet 1:1200–1201, 1965.
10. Shore JM, Morgenstern L, Berci G: An improved rigid choledoscope. Am J Surg 122:567–568, 1971.
11. Shore JM, Berci G: Choledochoscopy. In: Endoscopy Berci G (ed), New York, Appleton-Century-Crofts, 1976, p283–293.
12. Leslie DL: The use of choledochoscope. Med J Aust 1:236–237, 1962.
13. Reitsma BJ: Common duct stones (Thesis) Maastricht, University of Limburg Press, 1981.
14. Berci G, Shore JM, Morgenstern L, Hamlin JA: Choledochoscopy and operative fluoro-cholangiography. World J Surg 2:411–427, 1978.
15. Nora PF, Berci G, Dorazio RA, Kirshenbaum G, Shore JM, Tompkins PK, Wilson SD: Operative choledochoscopy. AM J Surg 133:105–110, 1977.
16. Berci G, Shore JM: Operative biliary endoscopy. In: Operative Biliary Radiology. Berci G, Hamlin JA (eds), Baltimore, Williams & Wilkins, 1981, p 169–185.
17. Feliciano DV, Mattox KL, Jordan GL: The value of choledochoscopy in exploration of the CBD. Ann Surg 191:649–654, 1980.
18. Rattner DW, Warshaw AL: Impact of choledochoscopy on the management of choledocholithiasis. Ann Surg 194:76–79, 1981.
19. Hamlin JA: Biliary ductal anomalies. In: Operative Biliary Radiology. Berci G, Hamlin JA (eds), Baltimore, Williams & Wilkins, 1981, p 120–125.
20. Wiechel KL: Surgical anatomy of the bile ducts. In: Opera-

tive biliary radiology. Berci G, Hamlin JA (eds), Baltimore, Williams & Wilkins, 1981, p 37–50.

21. Schein CJ, Hurwitt ES: The role of biliary tract endoscopy in clinical practice. Arch Surg 84:511–514, 1962.

22. Longland CJ: Choledochoscopy in choledocholithiasis. Brit J Surg 60:626–628, 1973.

23. Ottinger L.W, Warshaw AL, Bertlett MK: Intraoperative endoscopic evaluation of bile ducts. Am J Surg 127:465–468, 1974.

24. Griffin WT: Choledochoscopy. Am J Surg 132:697–698, 1976.

25. Finnis D, Rowntree T: Choledochoscopy in exploration of common bile duct. Brit J Surg 64:661–664, 1977.

26. Ashby BS: Choledochoscopy. Clin Gastroent 7:685–700, 1978.

27. Fourtanier G, LaCroix A, Escat J: L'intret de la choledocoscopie au cours de l'exploration de la voie biliaire principale pour lithiase. An Chir 32:122–125, 1978.

28. Kappas A, Alexander-Williams J, Keighley MRB, Watts GT: Operative choledochoscopy. Brit J Surg 66:177–179, 1979.

29. Botticher R, Knoch M: Diagnostischer und therapeutischer Stellenwert der intraoperativen Choledochoskopie. Langenb Arch 351:17–22, 1980.

30. Lennert K: Choledochoskopie Heidelberg, Springer, 1980.

31. Yap PC, Atacador M, Yap AG, Yap RG: Choledochoscopy as a complimentary procedure to operative cholangiography in biliary surgery. Am J Surg 140:648–652, 1980.

32. Motson RW, Wood AJ, DeJode LR: Operative choledochoscopy. Experience with the rigid choledochoscope. Brit J Surg 67:406–409, 1980.

33. Bauer JJ, Salky BA, Gelernt IM, Kreel I: Experience with the flexible fiberoptic choledochoscope. Ann Surg 194:161–166, 1981.

34. Kappes SK, Adams MB, Wilson SD: Intraoperative biliary endoscopy. Arch Surg 117:603–607, 1982.

35. DenBesten L, Berci G: Analysis of biliary surgery. A multi-institutional study organized by the International Biliary Association. In press.

36. Cedars-Sinai Medical Center (CSMC) Biliary (stone) cases. 1981–83. Surgical Staff Experience. Prepared for publication.

37. Saltzstein EC: Operative choledochoscopy and the retained common duct stone. (Editorial) Current Surgery, Nov-Dec, 371–373, 1981.

38. Iseli A, Marshall VC: Choledochoscopy: A comparison of a rigid and a flexible fiberoptic instrument. Med J Aust I:131–133, 1978.

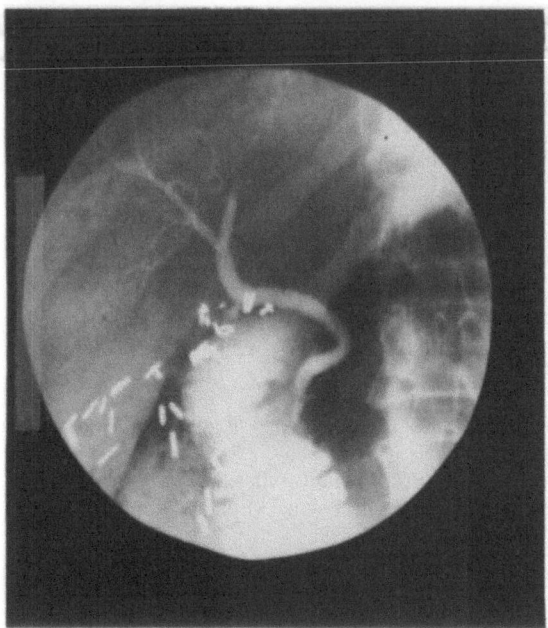

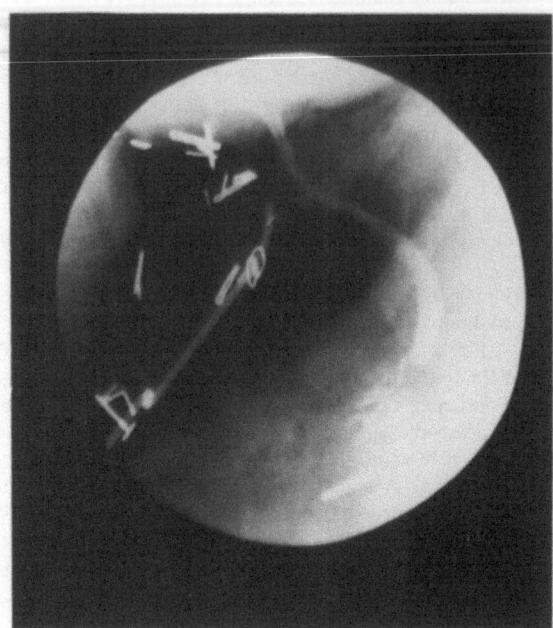

Fig. 5.1a. With this extreme curvature the surgeon is aware of the necessity not only to mobilize the duodenum but to keep it on a maximum stretch otherwise endoscopy of the distal duct will be difficult if not impossible.

Fig. 5.1b. An interesting 'lateral' short intramural segment of the sphincter region.

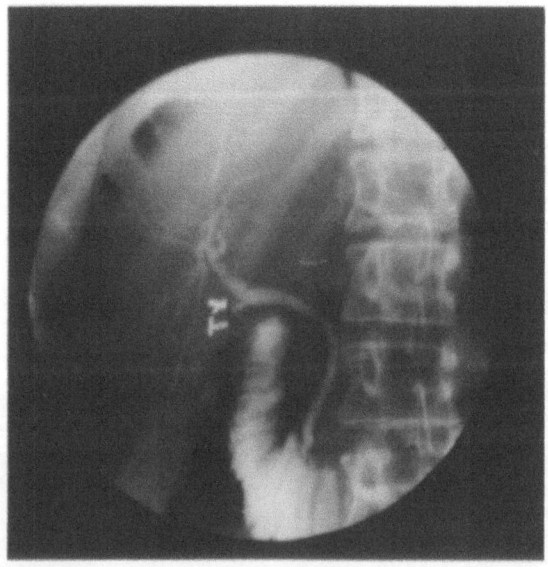

Figs. 5.1a–c. An initial cholangiogram is of importance to obtain information about the anatomy and configuration of the extra-hepatic biliary system before the duct is opened or endoscopy is performed.

Fig. 5.1c. The low entry of the CBD into the third part of the duodenum is not uncommon. In this case not only the generous mobilization of the duodenum has to be kept in mind, but also the site of the incision in the CBD (as near as possible to the duodenum). The longer (rigid) scope has to be used or in case of the flexible, it can be difficult to apply torque.

This topographical information is of importance to set up the tactics of the procedure and be aware of expected problems.

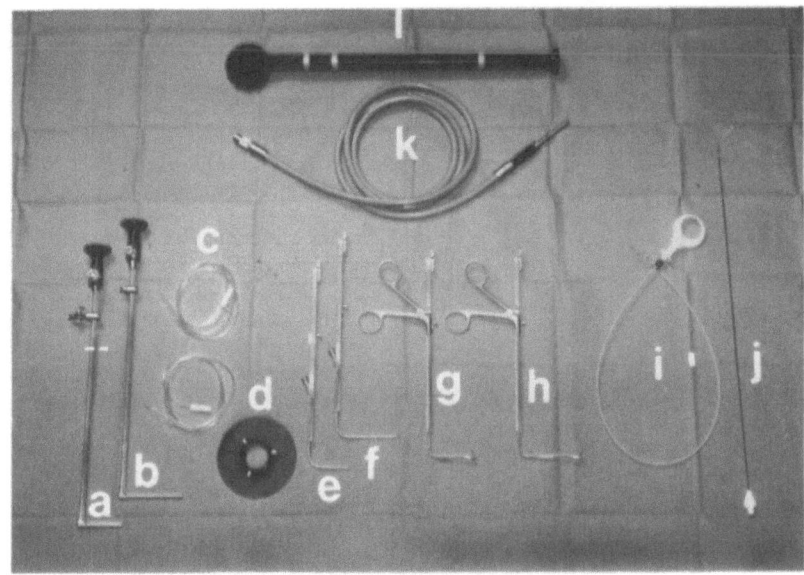

Fig. 5.2. The cholangioscope set. It should be prepared on a separate table and not mixed with the surgical hand instruments. Check the list of accessories and function before starting (Manufacturer: K. Storz Endoscopy Co., Tuttlingen, FRG).

(a) Cholangioscope with 40 mm horizontal limb. This scope is sufficient in the majority of cases.

(b) Same as above but with 60 mm horizontal limb. In cases with a longer distal duct (see Fig. 5.1a–c), this type will be more suitable.

(c) Two venous extension tubes.

(d) Clip on disc. Protects sterile manipulations (accidental touch of unsterile mask with sterile gloves).

(e and f) Instrument (accessory) guide channels for both sized scopes.

(g and h) Attachable stone grasping forceps. Very useful in impacted distal calculi.

(i) Dormia stone basket. Introduced through guide channel (e–f). Stone entrapment is performed under visual control.

(j) Fogarty Fr. 4 balloon catheter. Also introduced under visual control (e–f).

(k) Fiber optic light carrier bundle.

(l) Rigid teaching attachment. Removal of calculi is a teamwork and needs simultaneous observation (surgeon and assistant) and precise coordination.

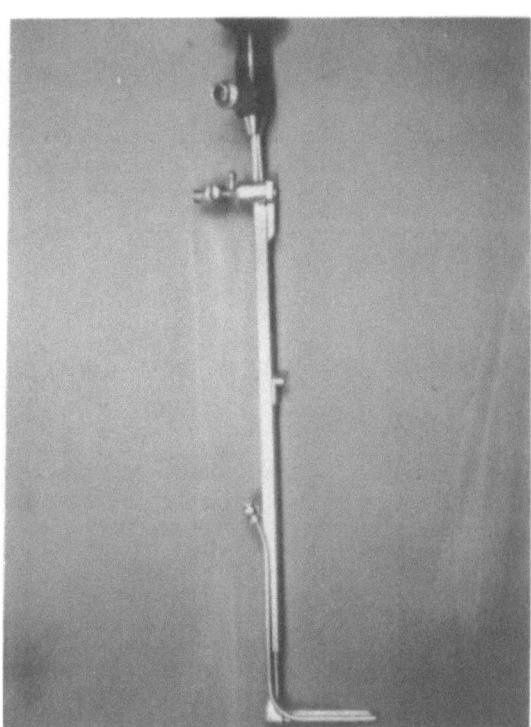

Fig. 5.3. A small instrument guide channel attached to the scope. If stones are seen it is worthwhile to remove them under visual control with the accessories mentioned under Figure 5.2i and j.

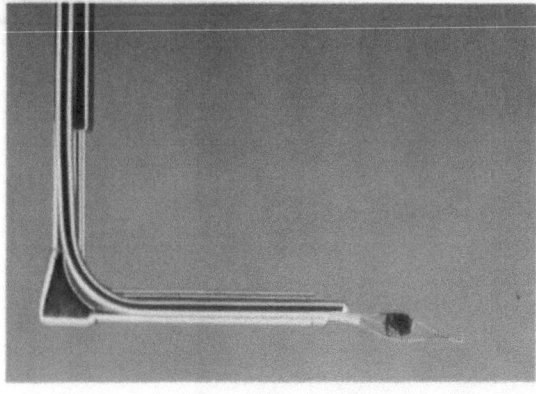

Fig. 5.4. The Dormia basket introduced through the instrument guide channel. The stone is entrapped under visual control. It is much faster to recover a calculus by endoscopy, than to withdraw the scope and attempt extraction with standard forceps. Removing the scope and reintroducing it, the ideal position is lost and many other factors (respiration, movements) can play a role in a delay or frustration. The instrument channel should be attached immediately.

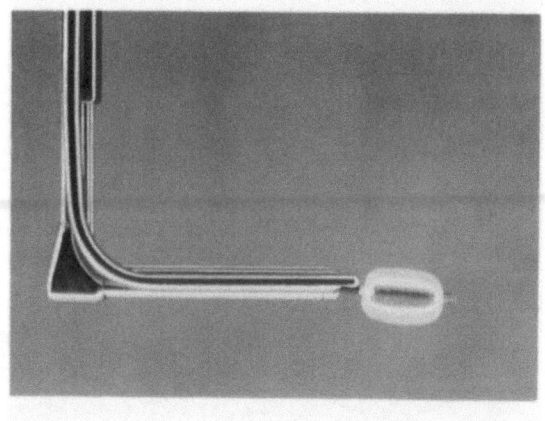

Fig. 5.5. The same instrument channel, but this time the Fr. 4 balloon catheter is advanced. If the calculus is seen the tip of the catheter, including the balloon, is forwarded beyond the stone, inflated and withdrawn together with the stone. It is very useful in hepatic stones, but it is also an important maneuver in the distal duct where previously biliary balloon catheters were advanced blindly into the duodenum, inflated and palpated. During withdrawal the balloon had to be deflated to pass the sphincter, but the degree of desufflation was not controlled *because it was not seen.* Therefore, it was a very common phenomenon for the balloon during the deflation to suddenly jump through the sphincter area and a smaller calculus was bypassed. The same procedure can now be performed under precise visual control. The balloon is advanced through the sphincter, inflated, and withdrawn, and desufflated under visual control and reinflated as necessary.

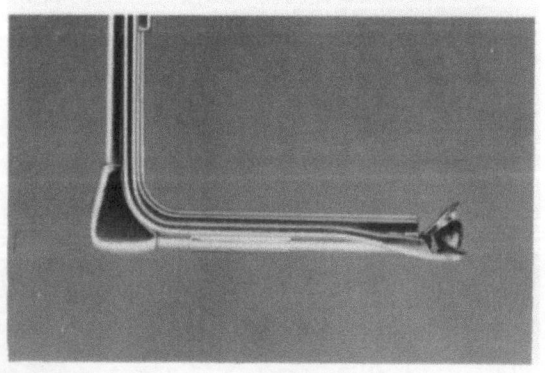

Fig. 5.6. The attached stone forceps has the advantage that it moves together with the instrument. In impacted stones, it is of great advantage to have an instrument which moves together with the vision and can be controlled with one hand. The other hand keeps the duodenum on a stretch to facilitate vision. Proper position of the forceps with the open jaws. The stone can be crushed or retrieved.

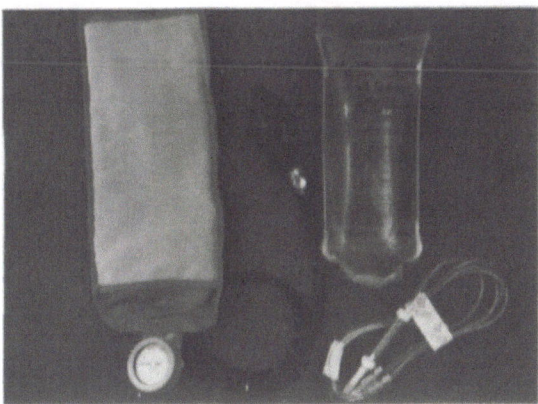

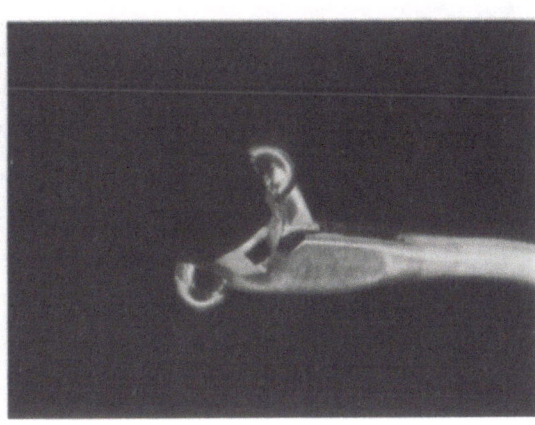

Fig. 5.7. Due to an extremely small irrigating channel a Fenwall pressure bag is used (200 mm Hg). This will provide a stream to irrigate, clean out the debris or blood, and dilate the duct. Because of the great resistance of this tube, the water pressure in the duct will be within the acceptable range.

Fig. 5.8. Attachable biopsy forceps. If suspicious areas are seen a forceps can be attached and tissue samples can be taken. It is very important in staging tumors.

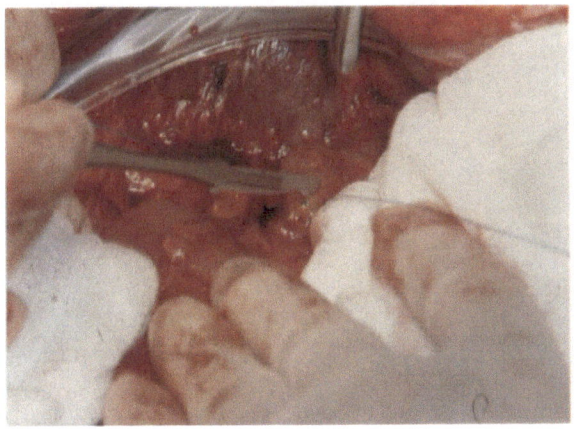

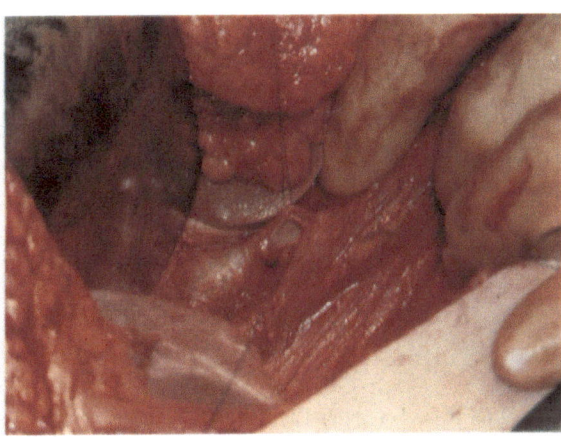

Fig. 5.9. After the CBD is verified, stay sutures are inserted which elevate the anterior wall and a small incision (10 mm) is made. The site of the incision should be carefully selected according to the anatomy and the length of the distal duct.

Fig. 5.10. The incision in the anterior wall is kept open with stay sutures which facilitate the introduction of the cholangioscope.

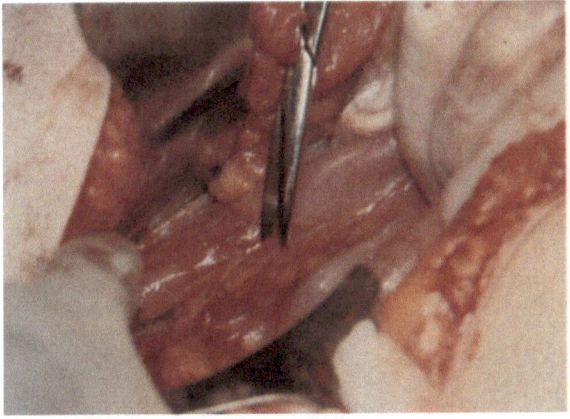

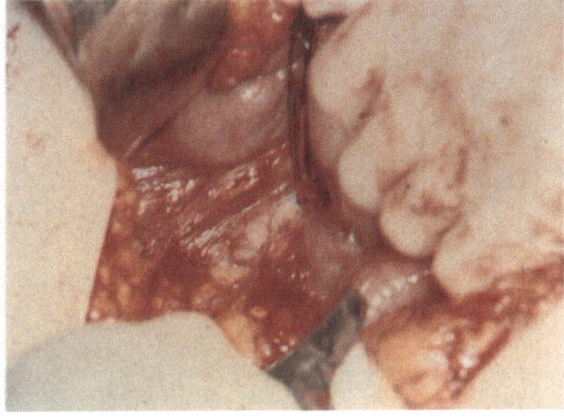

Fig. 5.11. If the cystic duct cholangiogram is positive and the CBD has to be explored (or a stone can be palpated), the most important step before opening the duct, is *to mobilize the duodenum*

Fig. 5.12. No operative biliary endoscopy should ever be performed without a generous mobilization (Kocher maneuver) because this is the most important step. It is done initially but sharp dissection.

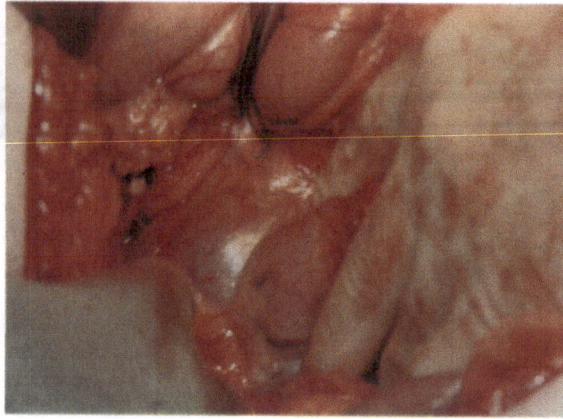

Fig. 5.13. and continued with blunt dissection according to the anatomy of the structures.

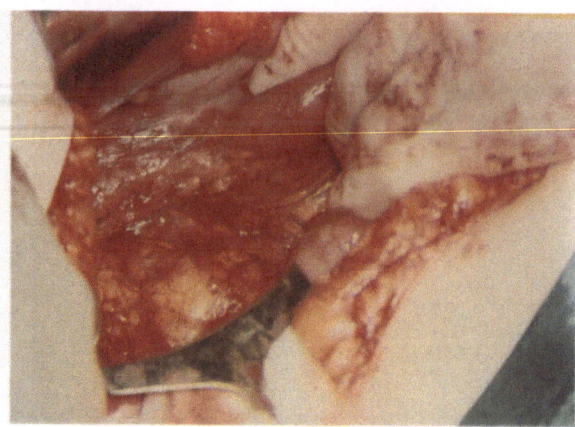

Fig. 5.14. The entire second and third part of the duodenum should be seen. The peritoneal fold should be mobilized distally as far as possible.

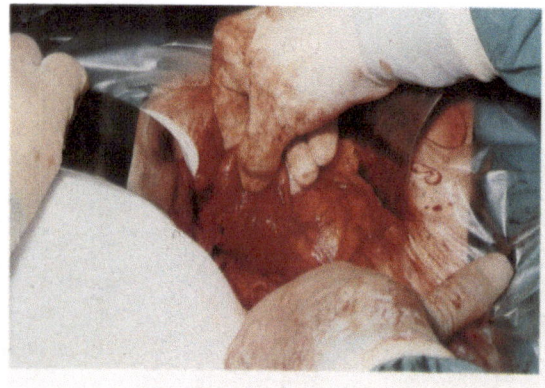

Fig. 5.15. In case of optimal mobilization of the duodenum, you can stretch even a long and tortuous duct in addition to palpation of the area.

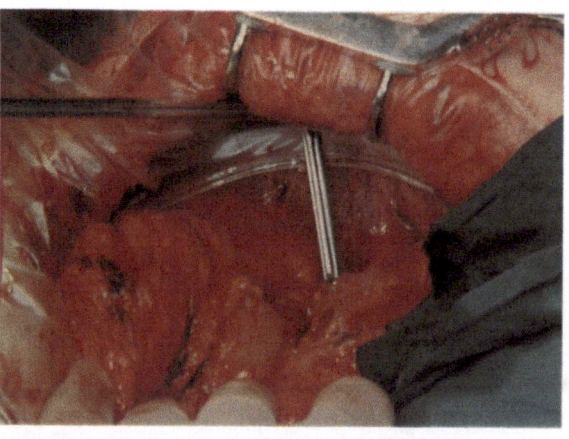

Figs. 5.16a–d. For orientation, the patient's leg or distal duct is on your left side. The surgeon operates from the patient's right. Photographs were taken from the patient's left side.
Fig. 5.16a. The cholangioscope is checked before introduction in respect to illumination and irrigation. It is of paramount importance that a CBD exploration should never be performed with a small skin incision or without proper exposure.

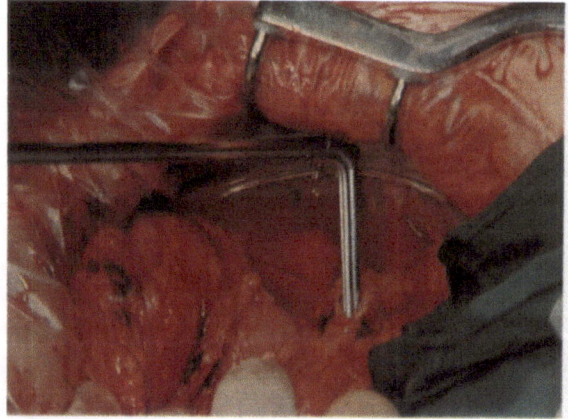

Fig. 5.16b. The scope is gently introduced and then turned towards the assumed direction. It is very important to avoid brisk movements. As soon as resistance is felt the position of the tip has to be changed. If there are any difficulties, remove the scope and probe the direction of the duct and reintroduce the instrument again.

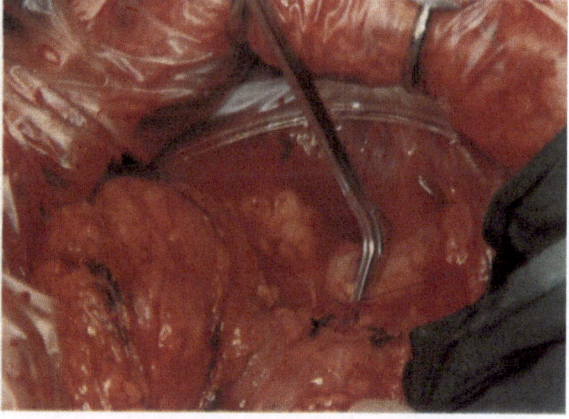

Fig. 5.16c. If the scope is introduced into the duct and you are looking through, you will first see a red or yellowish disc. This means that the tip of the telescope is touching the wall.

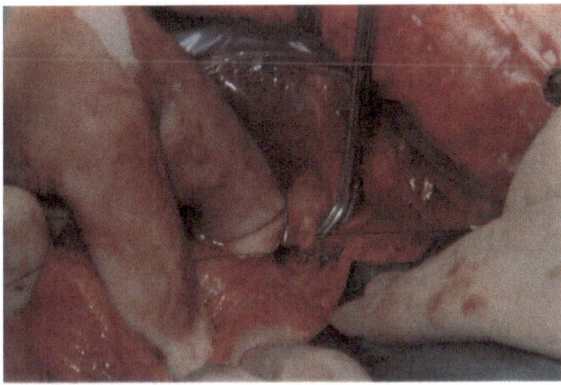

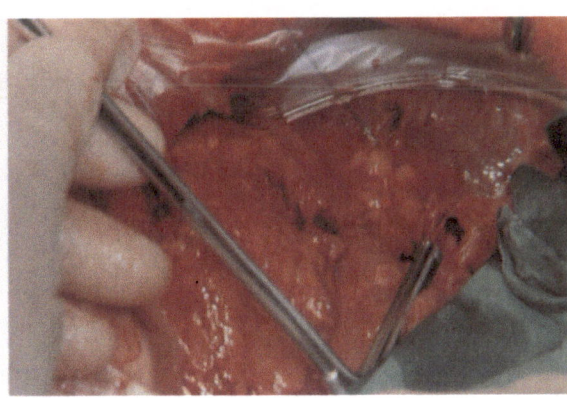

Fig. 5.16d. The most important maneuver is that the operator with one hand grasps the mobilized duodenum. You can palpate with the index finger the position of the scope and apply traction. Looking through the red and/or yellow disc will disappear and the duct will come into vision. If this maneuver does not help, withdraw the scope slightly, but keep the duodenum on traction and the lumen will be visible. As soon as you can see the interior of the duct, you can advance now under visual control.

Fig. 5.18a. The scope is now turned around 180° and is introduced towards the hepatic bifurcation. The stay sutures are held on a stretch. As soon as the tip with the saline stream disappears into the lumen, the stay sutures are crossed to decrease leakage of irrigating fluid.

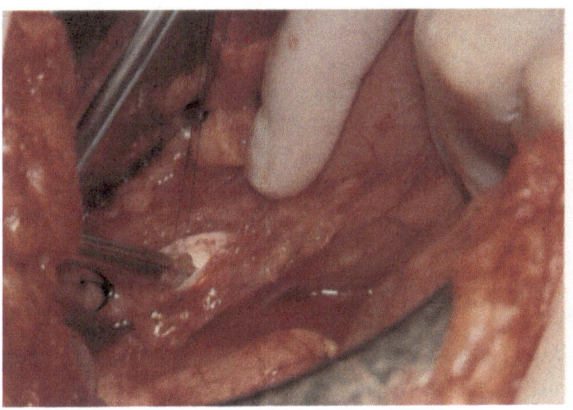

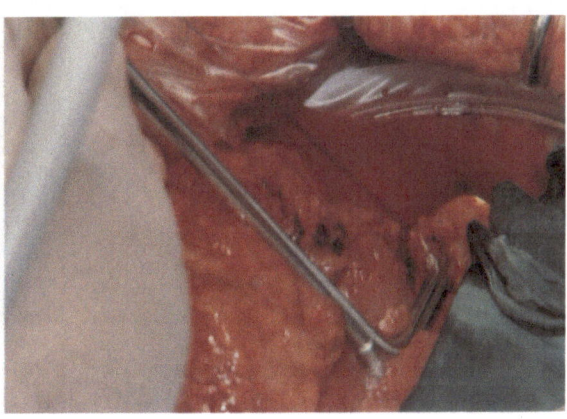

Fig. 5.17a. This is another patient. For information the patient's feet (distal duct) are on your right. The scope is slowly introduced.

Fig. 5.18b. The scope is further advanced into the proximal duct. This is a much simpler maneuver than endoscopic inspection of the distal duct. As soon as the bifurcation comes into vision, the individual orifices (right and left) can be observed.

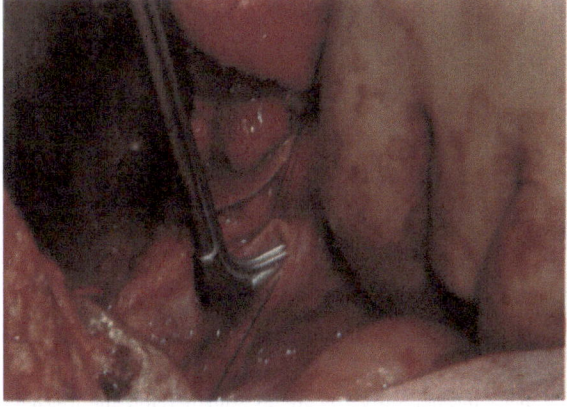

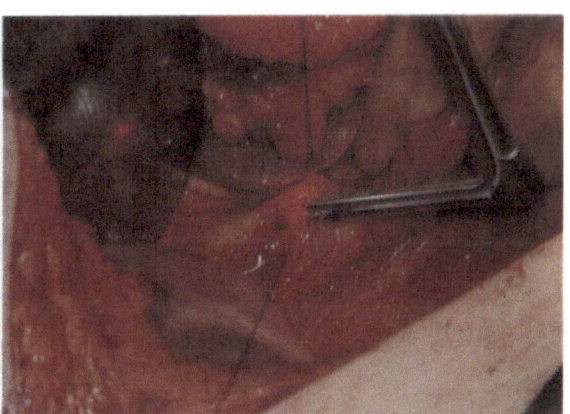

Fig. 5.17b. The same patient as Figure 5.17a and the same position, but the scope is further introduced towards the sphincter area. Note that the other hand of the operator palpates and stretches the duct with the mobilized duodenum in front of the tip of the scope.

Fig. 5.19a. The scope is introduced into the proximal duct in another patient after the stay sutures are lifted. The distal duct can be kept on a gentle stretch.

68

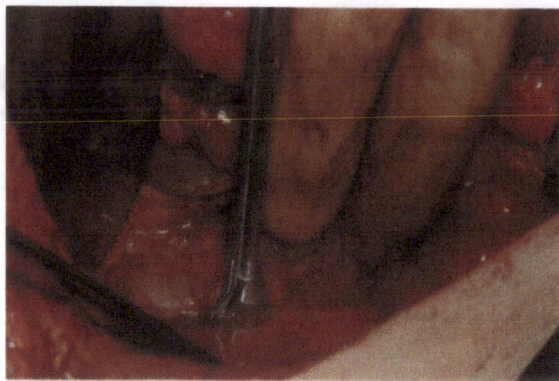

Fig. 5.19b. Same patient as displayed in Figure 5.19a, but the scope is introduced in one of the main branches.

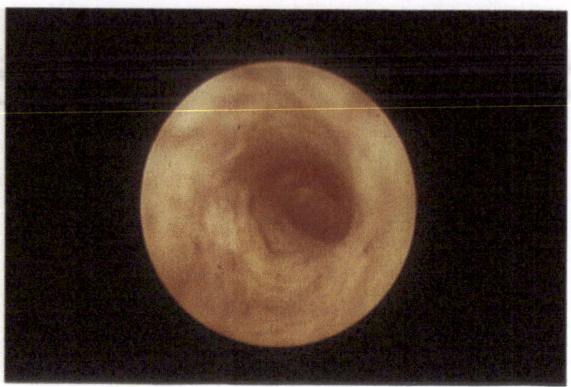

Fig. 5.20a. Endoscopic view of a normal appearing distal duct with the sphincter slightly obscured at a 6 o'clock position. This area should be observed for a longer period with irrigation to obtain a view of the sphincter in the open and closed positions. It can have various shapes and configurations (for details see text).

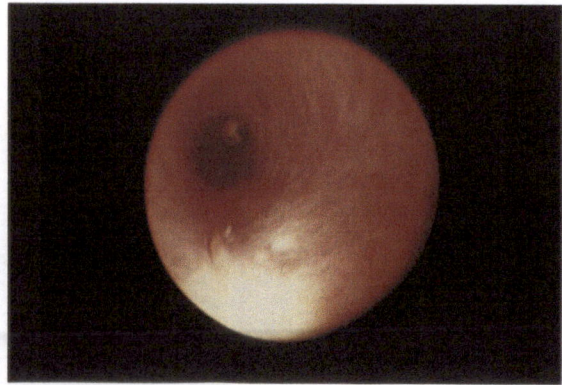

Fig. 5.20b. Endoscopic view of the distal duct with a slight inflammed wall (cholangitis). The closed sphincter at the very end is seen.

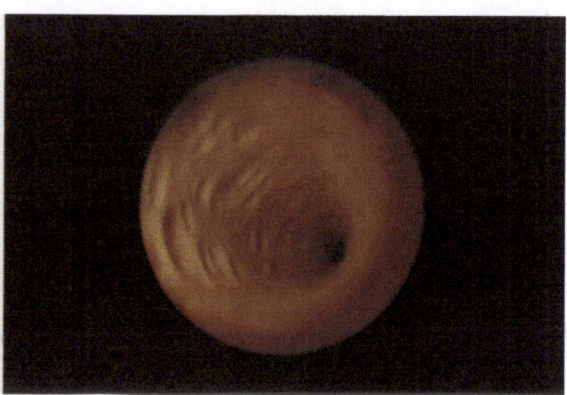

Fig. 5.20c. Distal duct with cholangitis as seen through the endoscope. The sphincter is in the open position.

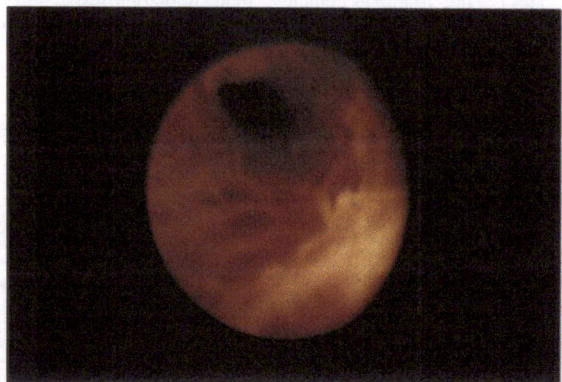

Fig. 5.20d. A more severe cholangitis with debris and wide open sphincter. The sphincter has to be seen under all conditions to make sure that this area is endoscopically well inspected. The advancement of a Fr. 4 Fogarty balloon catheter through the instrument channel, passing the sphincter and inflating and deflating, under visual control, can be of help. In difficult cases it is of utmost importance to make sure that stones are not overlooked.

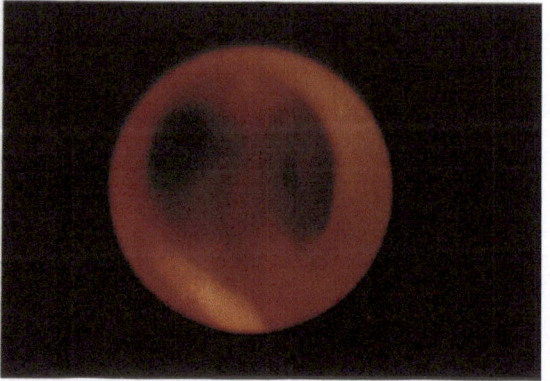

Fig. 5.21a. Endoscopic view of the main bifurcation. Moderate cholangitis. Small branches draining into the left duct (on your right). The anatomy varies greatly, and therefore the area has to be inspected according to the findings (appearances of orifices). If the situation is unclear withdraw the scope until the main bifurcation comes into vision, and then advance it further under endoscopic control.

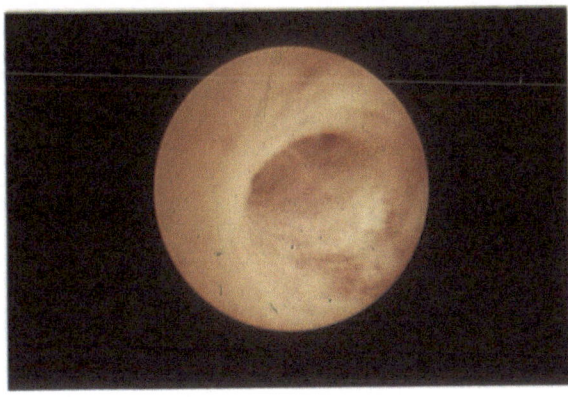

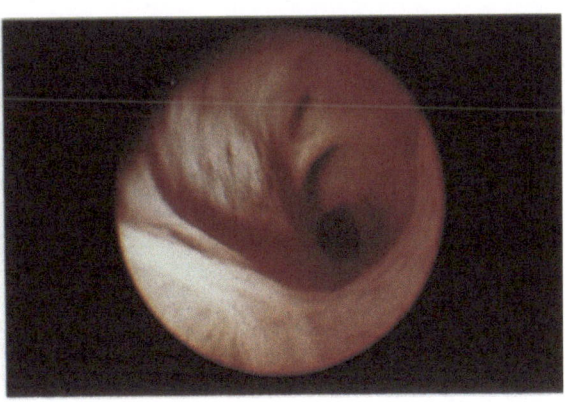

Fig. 5.21b. Bifurcation in a normal looking duct. If cholangitis is present, it first affects the distal duct. The common hepatic or major hepatic branches are not as frequently involved as the choledochus.

Fig. 5.21c. Cholangitic appearance of a hepatic trifurcation.

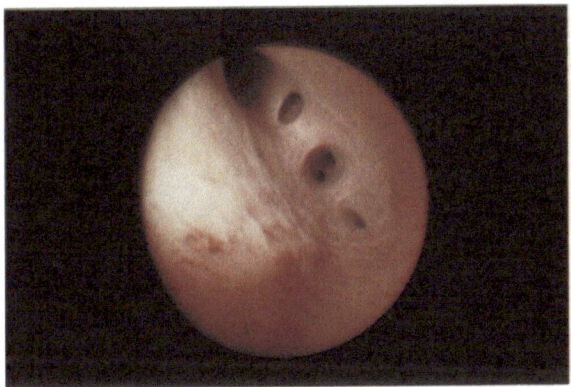

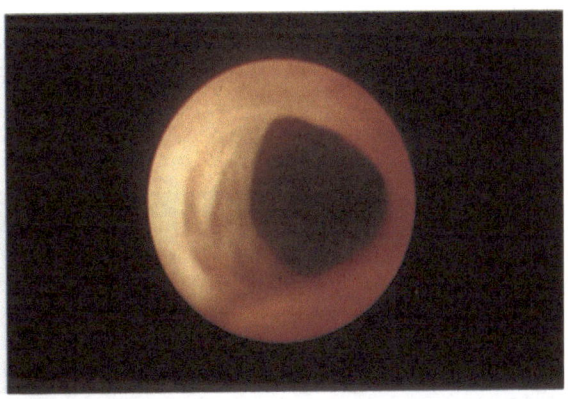

Fig. 5.21d. A slight hyperaemia in the intraparenchymal distribution of orifices. Even tertiary bifurcations can be well seen.

Fig. 5.22a. Floating stone in the common hepatic duct in front of the bifurcation.

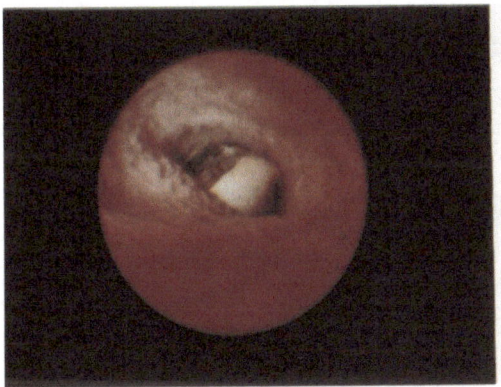

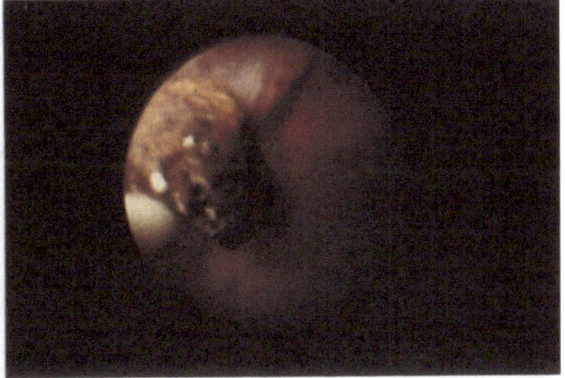

Fig. 5.22b. Impacted stone in the distal duct with cholangitis. There are the cases where manipulation can be performed more precisely under visual control. You may try to dislodge a stone with a balloon catheter passing beyond a stone and bringing the stone into the incision, or using the attachable stone forceps, it can be grasped and removed. The Dormia basket can also be applied. It depends on the dilatation and appearance of the duct. During the inspection you gain the impression: is the wall thick, rigid or soft? You may select your manipulating accessories accordingly.

Fig. 5.22c. Floating stone in front of the bifurcation.

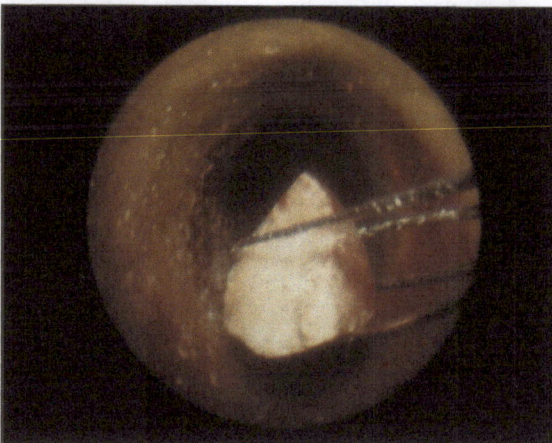

Fig. 5.23a. The Dormia basket is applied by advancing it through the instrument channel *beyond the stone and opened up*. During withdrawal the basket is manipulated with the instrument to entrap the calculus between the wires. The basket is slightly closed by the assistant whereby the operator, during the same period, slightly advances the sheath of the basket to keep the stone in one position. The stone in the basket including instrument, are withdrawn together.

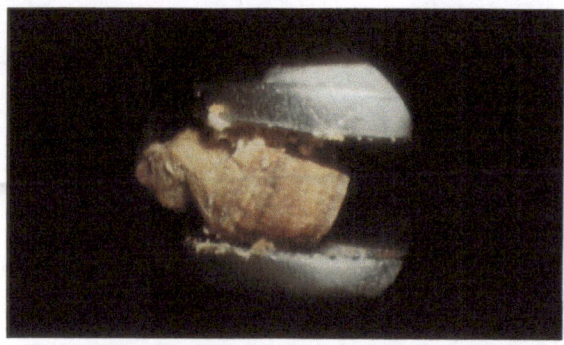

Fig. 5.23b. The attached forceps grasping an impacted stone as seen through the endoscope.

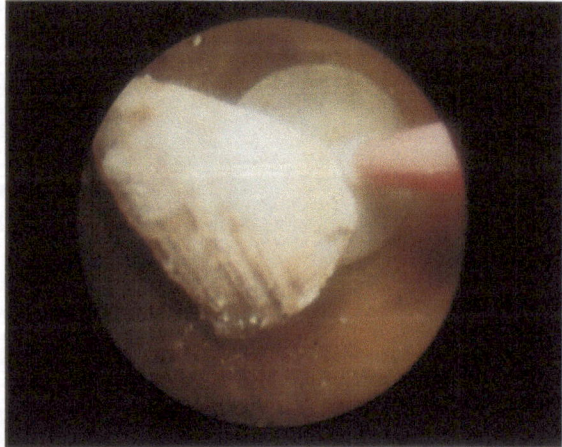

Fig. 5.23c. The inflated balloon catheter which was advanced beyond the stone and inflated, is withdrawn together.

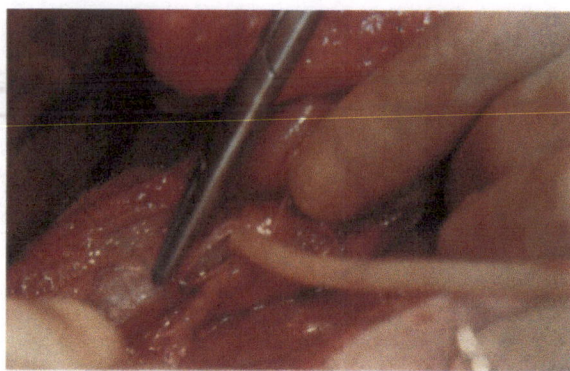

Fig. 5.24a. Always insert a large T-tube (Fr. 16–18) with a short horizontal limb.

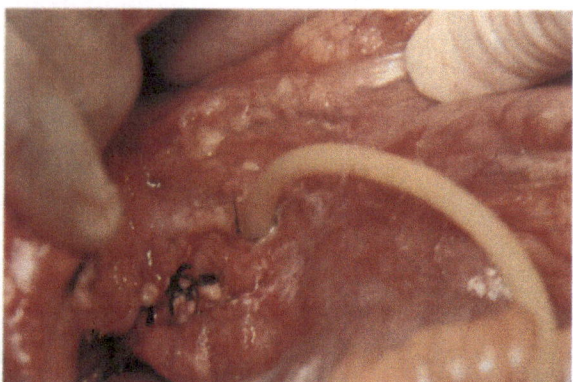

Fig. 5.24b. After closure of the incision around the T-tube you may check for a water tight seal.

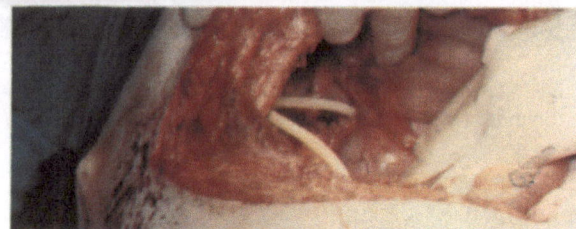

Fig. 5.24c. Do not loop the T-tube. If the abdomen is open you can pull the tube gently and carefully to straighten it out somehow and exit it through the flank.

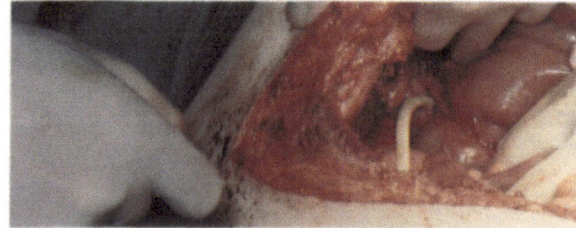

Fig. 5.24d. You should have made only a slight curvature. (Never bring out the tube in the midline or in the incision.)

Despite the most efficient technique, it can occur that a stone can be missed. If a relatively large T-tube is inserted in a proper configuration a retained stone(s) can be retrieved in the postoperative period through the T-tube tract, with a 90 to 95% success rate. It is the safest and fastest corrective measure for removal of missed calculi (for details see Chapter 8 Postoperative Removal of Retained Stones Through the T-tube Tract).

CHAPTER 6

BILIARY MANOMETRY AND DEBIMETRY

1. Introduction

Despite its introduction some 45 years ago, biliary manometry is not an established per-operative procedure during surgical intervention on the biliary tract. Moreover the techniques available for measuring various indices of pressure within the biliary tract lack standardization and despite a wealth of retrospective reported experience (1–6), there have been no prospective clinical trials designed to evaluate the diagnostic accuracy of mano-debimetric indices. It is difficult therefore to define the indications for operative manometry. Indeed some would consider the procedure as unnecessary and misleading. Against this are good and carefully documented reports which demonstrate that biliary pressure and flow studies complement per-operative cholangiography such that the predictive value of their combination exceeds that of either investigation alone.

2. Usage

Biliary manometry and/or debimetry (flow rate through the papillary orifice at a standard pressure head) have been used in the following circumstances:

(i) In lieu of or in the absence of facilities for cholangiography, primarily to detect common bile duct calculi and the need for exploration of the CBD. Irrespective of claims to the contrary, there is little doubt that biliary debimetry is a poor substitute for cholangiography in this respect since calculi may be present with normal pressure indices and flow rate. When the sum of the area of the interstices between ductal calculi is equal to or exceeds 3 mm², the bile flow remains within the normal range (7).

(ii) In conjunction with per-operative cholangiography. This is practised by the author with a transducer/image intensifier system designed to provide synchronous combined cholangiomanometry. White and Bordley (6) reported a 1.0% incidence of recurrent gallstones 6 to 8 years after manometric cholangiography.

(iii) Selective use in suspected sphincter pathology usually in patients undergoing surgery for recurrent symptoms after cholecystectomy. In this instance operative biliary manometry may provide useful information to the surgeon and help to differentiate between organic stenosis and functional spasm.

(iv) Pharmacological studies to investigate the effect of hormones, peptides and pharmaceutical agents on the sphincter of Oddi. However, it seems likely that endoscopic manometry during ERCP with a special tri-lumen perfused catheter (8, 9) in the conscious patient will be used in the future to study drug and hormonal effects.

3. Pharmacology of the sphincter of Oddi (SO)

3.1. Effect of hormones and peptides

Cholecystokinin (CCK). This is the main stimulus to gallbladder contraction in response to a meal and CCK administration increases gallbladder pressure, decreases resistance through the SO and enhances bile flow (10). The activity of CCK depends on the COO H-terminal heptapeptide, a sequence found in gastrin which has a cholecystokinetic activity which is 1/15 that of CCK. Gastrin has no effect on the biliary pressure of cholecystectomized patients.

Glucagon. This hormone has a relaxant effect on

both the gallbladder musculature and the SO in man and has been shown to be an effective agent in the relief of biliary colic (12).

Secretin does not appear to have a significant cholecystokinetic effect in the human. Its effects on the gallbladder and SO musculature show considerable interspecies variation.

Caerulein. This is a peptide of similar composition to CCK extracted from amphibian skin. It has a marked cholecystokinetic effect about 3 times that induced by CCK. Both the gallbladder contraction and reduced resistance of SO are produced by a direct action on the smooth muscle. The synthetic peptide ceruletide has been shown to relieve the pain in biliary colic and we have observed a pronounced relaxant effect on the SO when the drug is administered intravenously during operative biliary manometry.

3.2. Effect of pharmacological agents
The drugs which decrease the resistance of the SO and thereby enhance bile flow through the papillary orifice are atropine, scopolamine, isoproterinol adrenalin, amylnitrite and glyceryl nitrite.

Drug induced spasm of the sphincter of Oddi is caused by morphine, pethidine, mecholyl and phenylephrine.

4. Biliary pressure indices

4.1. resting (initial, interdigestive) pressure
This fasting pressure ensures patency of the extrahepatic conduit and is a function of the hepatic secretory pressure and the contractile activity of the sphincteric musculature. Its value in the normal state is 6.4 ± 4.3 mmHg. As far as operative manometry is concerned, the term resting pressure should be confined to the measurement of the CBD pressure before the instillation of saline or contrast medium into the system. The level of the resting pressure has little or no predictive value in the diagnosis of obstructive CBD lesions including ductal calculi (14).

4.2. Passage (yield, opening) presssure
This is defined as the pressure head needed to overcome the resistance of the SO resulting in the passage of contrast material or saline into the duodenum. The normal range is 14–18 mmHg. The passage pressure is generally higher in patients with functional or organic obstruction at the sphincter region and in the presence of ductal calculi but the overlap with the normal range is such as to render this pressure index a poor predictor of obstructive disease in the individual case.

4.3. Filling pressure curves
These curves represent a dynamic and continuous pressure profile of the bile duct before, during and after constant pump injection of isotonic saline at the rate of 5 to 6 ml/min. Three types are encountered, I, II III (15) (Fig. 6.1). Type I outlines the normal situation and demonstrates contraction waves due to sphincter activity. Although the pressure rises during infusion, there is no residual pressure after injection (Fig. 6.2).

In Type II (Fig. 6.3) there is a gradual increase of the pressure during infusion, absence of sphincteric wave contractions and a residual pressure after injection. This pressure profile indicates functional (spasm) or organic obstruction of the sphincteric region. The two can be differentiated by repeating the pressure profile after the administration of CCK or ceruletide, both agents result in a lowering of the pressure during pump infusion and abolition of a residual pressure in cases of functional obstruction. Type II pressure filling curve which remains unaltered after CCK or ceruletide does not differentiate papillary stenosis from papillary oedema or impacted calculi at the lower end of the CBD. The long term outcome of patients with this type II pressure filling curve in whom the operative cholangiogram did not show any abnormality have demonstrated presistent symptoms and episodes of cholangitis which necessitated re-exploration in some 30 to 35% of patients (16).

In some patients with an otherwise normal operative cholangiogram, the pressure in the CBD generated during pump injection barely exceeds the perfusion pressure due to pump delivery and intrinsic resistance to flow of the tubing. In addition phasic sphincter activity is absent and the CBD pressure before and after pump injection is low (Type III – Fig. 6.4). We have interpreted these manometric findings as indicative of hypotonia and indeed it is difficult to outline the intrahepatic biliary tree during operative cholangiography because of rapid and immediate passage of contrast medium into the duodenum. The full significance of this state is uncertain but some patients have developed relapsing attacks of acute pancreatitis presumably due to duodeno-pancreatic reflux.

4.4. Residual pressure

This is defined as a sustained rise in the CBD after injection. The exact reading depends on rate of injection but in general a residual pressure is unequivocally present if the post injection pressure exceeds the initial or resting pressure by 2 mmHg (Fig. 6.5).

4.5. Flow rate (debimetry)

This is measured by gravimetric (hydrostatic) techniques such as the Caroli's instrument or the syringe barrel technique (17) usually with the reservoir held at a vertical height of 30 cm above the CBD. The normal range is a flow rate above 12 to 16 ml/min. In our experience this test is a poor predictor of obstructive disease. It is found abnormally low in 30% of patients with an otherwise normal biliary tree and the flow rate is normal in 30% of patients with obvious ductal pathology (calculi) at cholangiography (Fig. 6.6).

4.6. Incremental pressure and recovery time

These indices were introduced by Boeckl and Hell (18) and are obtained from the dynamic CBD filling pressure curve following rapid hand injection of approximately 10.0 ml of isotonic saline at a rate of 1.0 ml/sec. This technique is far better standardized with pump delivery as hand injection is extremely variable. The incremental pressure is defined as the rise in pressure above basal at the end of injection (normal range = 15.0 ± 1.0 mmHg). The time in seconds required for the pressure to reach initial pre-injection values is the recovery time (normal range 5.0 ± 0.5 sec).

5. Dynamic (transducer)manometry

It is the author's opinion that all gravimetric techniques (Caroli's instrument and disposable analogues, the syringe barrel technique and debimetry) are insufficiently accurate and rely on subjective end points for their interpretation. Biliary manometry *must be measured by indwelling or external transducers using an irrigating system with constant pump infusion of saline* with adequate calibration and an accurate assessment of the compliance of the system used. These criteria are as valid and essential in the monitoring of biliary pressure as they are in recordings of the oesophageal high pressure zone. Transducer techniques allow accurate monitoring of the biliary pressure both during ERCP and at operation during biliary tract surgery where the dynamic pressure profile of the CBD provides useful information regarding disorders of the sphincter of Oddi particularly during secondary biliary intervention.

5.1. Endoscopic sphincter zone activity

SO pressure activity has been measured during endoscopic retrograde cholangiographic pancreatography using both single-lumen and triple-lumen perfused catheters connected to external transducers (8, 9). The findings have shown a basal SO pressure similar to the resting CBD pressure and phasic SO contractions which in the normal state assume a predominantly antegrade direction. On the other hand, the direction of SO phasic activity in patients with CBD calculi is predominently retrograde (9).

5.2. Technique of operative biliary manometry

(a) Apparatus. The components include an infusion pump with an adjustable flow rate, external transducer, fine bore polyethylene tubing (1.0 mm internal diameter) connected to the CBD cannula and to the transducer and a pressure recorder (Fig. 6.7).

The delivery system consists of an infusion pump with an adjustable flow rate. We have observed from our experience that a flow rate of 6.0 ml per minute gives optimum and reproducible results. The syringe is filled with isotonic saline, mounted on the pump and connected by polyethylene tubing to a 3 way tap which leads to the pressure line and is also connected to the cannula to be inserted into the CBD. After calibration of the transducer (zero equals level of CBD) and elimination of air bubbles from the system, the pump is switched on and the pressure generated with the tip of the cannula held at the level of the CBD is measured and recorded. The corrected pressure during infusion with the cannula in the CBD can then be calculated by subtraction.

(b) Practical considerations. It is essential that all drugs known to affect sphincter activity are not administered to the patient within 60 min. of the procedure. All our patients have received endotracheal anaesthesia with muscle relaxants (D-tubocurarine). It is essential that manometry is undertaken at the outset before the anatomy is disturbed and after a minimum of dissection i.e., that required for insertion of the cannula via the cystic duct. It should also be performed before cholangiography. Good quality cholangiograms can be obtained by substituting the saline syringe with one containing Hypaque (Na diatrizoate, 20%) using the pump infusion system after the manometry has been completed. Retractors including self-retaining ones should not be in use during manometry and the peritoneal cavity, particularly the supracolic compartment, must be devoid of swabs or packs.

(c) Cannula. Several are available. Metal cannulae such as the Berci-Shore have several advantages – good design, ease of insertion and good flow characteristics. However it tends to distort the CBD by virtue of the weight of the cannula and its holding clamp. This disadvantage can be overcome if the holding clamp is carefully positioned and held by a suture to the edges of the wound. The one essential characteristic of a CBD cannula vis a vis its use for accurate manometry is *the presence of side holes*.

6. Disorders of the sphincter of Oddi

This remains a controversial area although there is now some consensus with regard to the existence of specific disorders, eg. stenosis. There is however no internationally accepted classification. A suggested classification which the author has found useful in clinical practice is shown in Table 6.1.

Table 6.1. Disorders of sphincter of Oddi

Iatrogenic stricture
Papillitis/oedema
Stenosis (Choledocho-duodenal junctional stenosis)
Functional disorders
(i) Hypertonic sphincter   (ii) Hypotonic sphincter

6.1. Iatrogenic stricture

This is a complication after CBD exploration resulting from the use (often forcible) of metal sounds which are passed via the choledochotomy into the duodenum to check patency or overcome a hold up of contrast visualised on the operative cholangiogram. This practice often results in the creation of false passage/fistula between the transpancreatic segment and the duodenum, pancreatic damage and postoperative pancreatitis. There is usually a latent period of 1 to 5 years before the patient presents with recurrent episodes of jaundice and fever. The stricture differs from that of papillary stenosis in that it affects the entire length of the trans-pancreatic segment (Fig. 6.8). In a series of 6 patients afflicted by this disorder, all had metal bouginage of the terminal bile duct during the first biliary intervention. Despite obvious deformity and narrowing of the proximal pancreatic duct, recurrent pancreatitis has not been a problem in these patients. Iatrogenic stricture of the lower end of the CBD is best avoided. There is nowadays no justification for blind metal instrumentation of this vulnerable region of the extrahepatic biliary tract. These patients are best treated by transection choledochoduodenostomy (19).

6.2. Papillitis/oedema

A transitory papillitis and oedema is common after exploration of CBD und undelies the need for T-tube drainage after stone extraction and instrumentation of the CBD including the passage of balloon catheters.

Elevated CBD pressure in patients with acute cholecystitis was first reported by Schein (20). In our practice of early cholecystectomy for acute cholecystitis, we have observed biliary hypertension in 29 out of 34 patients who underwent operative biliary manometry. Exploration of CBD and choledochoscopy in these patients has shown that in the majority this is due to oedema/papillitis. Whilst this may have been the result of a recently passed calculus in some of these cases, no such evidence could be accrued with any certainty in the majority of these cases. It would appear therefore that papillitis and oedema are very common accompaniments of acute cholecystitis and that in the majority, this is a self limiting disorder with resolution following cholecystectomy. It could however be argued that recurrent episodes of acute cholecystitis may result in chronic inflammation of both the gallbladder and the sphincter of Oddi region. This hypothesis requires further scrutiny.

6.3. Papillary stenosis (Choledocho-duodenal junctional stenosis)

The existence of the disorder is now generally accepted. In the vast majority of cases, diagnosis is made after a previous cholecystectomy because of persistence of symptoms with recurrent episodes of jaundice or cholecystitis. The criteria for diagnosis must include the following: a dilated CBD, biliary hypertension particularly a residual pressure after injection and absence of phasic sphincteric activity. Most authors have excluded cases with additional local pathology such as small ductal calculi in the ampullary region. On the other hand it is difficult to conceive of an organic distal obstructive condition without stasis and therefore ductal stone formation. This insistence on the absence of other local pathology accounts for the low incidence (<1.0%) in some reported series of patients undergoing biliary surgery for calculous disease. Other estimates of the incidence of the condition in patients undergoing biliary tract surgery vary from 4 to 10.7%. The author has encountered 16 patients with papillary stenosis out of a series of 561 patients undergoing biliary tract surgery (2.8%). Another 9 patients fulfilled the criteria but had in addition small ductal calculi. All have presented with recurrent symptoms some 1 to 10 years after cholecystectomy.

Eleven out of the 16 have been female, the mean age of the group at the time of presentation has been 57 with a range of 35 to 70 years. Radiologically the stenosis involves only the sphincteric region (Fig. 6.9). A frequent finding is a bulbous distention of the infundibulum. Histological examination of biopsies of the affected region obtained through the choledochoscope have shown a spectrum of changes, but the most common findings have been fibrosis, chronic cellular infiltrate and atrophy of the microvilli (Figs. 6. 10a and b). Other changes which have been reported include fibroglandular hyperplasia and less commonly adenomyosis (5).

Most advocate sphincteroplasty for this condition with or without division of the septum between the juxtaposed pancreatic and bile duct sphincters. It is impossible to evaluate the long term results of this procedure from the reported literature. In the author's opinion, a complete division of the sphincteric complex is technically impossible since the superior sphincter extends well into the pancreatic segment of the CBD. The procedure therefore results in incomplete division and may induce duodeno-pancreatic reflux and relapsing pancreatitis in some patients.

6.4. Functional disorders

Functional disorders of the sphincter of Oddi have been documented by both operative and ERCP manometry. Evidence of functional obstruction (spasm) relieved by spasmolytic agents is obtained in 20% of patients undergoing cholecystectomy with a normal operative cholangiogram (Type II pressure filling curve). In the author's experience this group exhibit a high incidence of persistent post-cholecystectomy symptoms and some are found subsequently to have ductal disease (ductal calculi, stenosis). It seems likely that the term biliary dyskinesia refers to this group of patients. It is possible that the functional disorder precedes the development of organic stenosis of the sphincteric region.

In a comparative study of sphincter of Oddi motor activity in patients with ductal calculi and controls, no difference in either the basal or phasic SO pressure was observed between the 2 groups (9). However in patients with ductal calculi the sphincteric contractions were predominantly retrograde whereas in the control group the majority of contractions occured in an antegrade direction. This abnormality may contribute to stasis and therefore stone formation or retention. Alternatively this abnormal motility may be secondary to

76

the ductal calculi. Obviously further studies are needed to establish the exact relationship between SO motor activity and bile duct calculi.

Finally there is a rare subgroup of patients in whom sphincter contractions are absent or weak and in whom the sphincter of Oddi offers little or no resistance to flow during pump perfusion of saline into the CBD via the cystic duct. In these patients it is difficult to outline the intra-hepatic biliary tree with contrast medium because of instantaneous egress into the duodenum on injection. These patients have a hypotonic sphincter which may result in duodeno-biliary/pancreatic reflux. The association of this condition with relapsing pancreatitis merits further investigation. The hypothesis which has been suggested involves the occurrence of abnormal segmental duodenal hyperactivity in some patients with chronic pancreatitis with reflux of duodenal contents through an incompetent sphincter into the pancreatic duct.

References

1. Caroli J: La radiomanomètrie biliare. Sem Hôp Paris 1946, 22:1985.
2. Albot G Oliver C, Liboude H: Radiomanometric evaluation of the biliary ducts. Experience with 418 cases. Gastroenterology 24:242, 1953.
3. Mallet-Guy P, Rose DF: Peroperative manometry and radiology in biliary tract disorders. Br J Surg 44:55, 1956.
4. Yvergneaux JP, Bauwens E, Yvergneaux E: Diagnostic de la sténose oddienne benigne dans une série homogène de 1150 interventions biliares serous radiomanomètrie. Ann Chir 28:545–552, 1974.
5. Boeckl O: Rationale for primary operations on the papilla of Vater. Eur Surg Res 8:400–410, 1976.
6. White TT, Bordley JN: One per cent incidence of recurrent gallstones six to eight years after manometric cholangiography. Ann Surg 188:562–569, 1978.
7. Barraya L, Pujol-Soler R, Yvergneaux JP: The sphincter of Oddi. Schematized anatomy. Coll Inter Digest, Chicago Meeting, 1974.
8. Carr-Locke DJ, Gregg JA: Endoscopic manometry of pancreatic and biliary sphincter zones in man: basal results in healthy volunteers. Dig Dis Sci 26:7–15, 1981.
9. Toouli J, Geenen JE, Hogan WJ, Dodds WJ, Arndorfer RC: Sphincter of Oddi motor activity: a comparison between patients with common bile duct stones and controls. Gastroenterology 82:111–117, 1982.
10. Sandblom PH, Voegtlin WL, Ivy AC: The effect of cholecystokinin on the choledochoduodenal mechanism (sphincter of Oddi). Am J Physiol 113:175–180, 1935.
11. Lin TM, Spray GF: Effect of pentagastrin, cholecystokinin, caerulein and glucagon on the choledochal resistance and bile flow of the conscious dog. Gastroenterology 56:1178, 1969.
12. Stower MJ, Foster GE, Hardcastle JD: A trial of glucagon in the treatment of painful biliary tract disease. Br J Surg 69:591–592, 1982.
13. Ganzina F, Santamaria A: Caerulein (Ceruletide). A review. Acta gastro-ent belg 39:169–185, 1976.
14. Cuschieri A: Intraoperative pressure measurements (biliary manometry) in: Operative Biliary Radiology. Berci G, Hamlin JA. Baltimore/London, Williams & Wilkins, 1981, p 187–196.
15. Cuschieri A, Howell Hughes J, Cohen M: Biliary pressure studies during cholecystectomy. Br J Surg 59:267–273, 1972.
16. Cuschieri A: Cholangiomanometry. Br J Surg 68:369–370, 1981.
17. Besançon F, Pironneaur A, Lopez-Macedo L, Longuet YL, Debray CH: Technique nouvelle et simple d'exploration opératoire du cholédoque: le débimètre à flotteur perfusé sous pression constante et élevée. Arch mal app dig 54:59–70, 1965.
18. Boeckl O, Hell E: Intraoperative gallenwegsdiagnostik mit radio-electro-manometrie. Dt med Wschr 92:1708, 1967.
19. Cuschieri A, Wood RAB, Metcalf MJ, Cumming JGR: Long term experience with transection choledochoduodenostomy. World J Surg 7:502–504, 1983.
20. Schein CJ: Post-cholecystectomy Syndromes – a Clinical Approach to Etiology, Diagnosis and Management. New York, Harper and Row, 1978.
21. Vayre P, Jost JL, Hureau J, Roux M: La sclérodystrophie oddienne. J Chir 115:489–496, 1978.

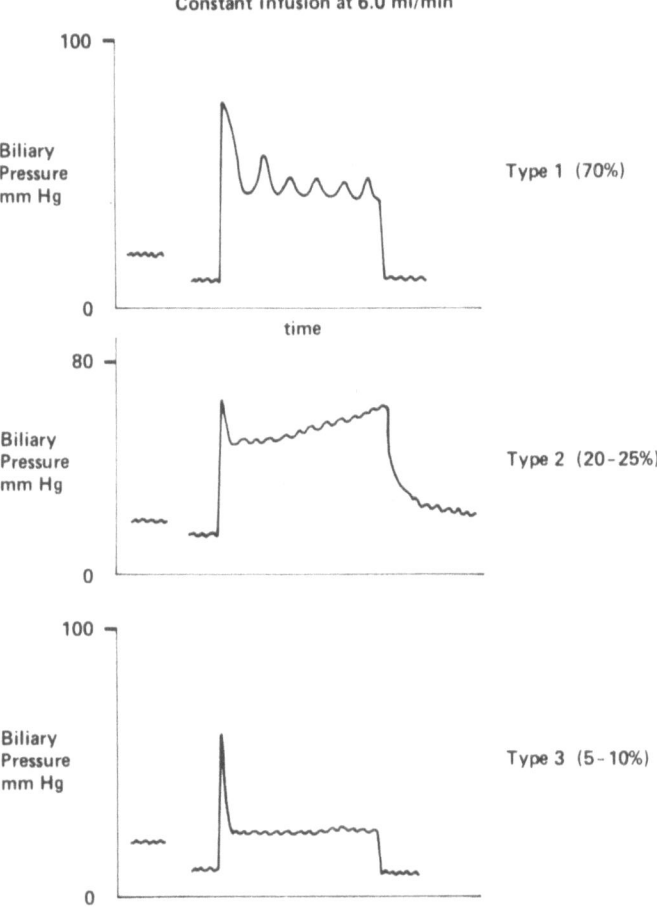

Fig. 6.1. Schematic representation of the 3 types of pressure filling curves.

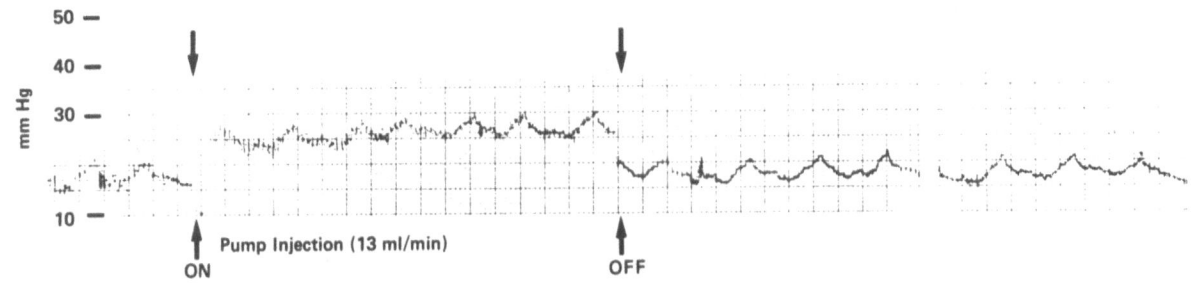

Fig. 6.2. Type I pressure filling curve. This is encountered in 70–75% of patients with normal operative cholangiography. It represents the normal situation. Phasic sphincter activity is outlined and the pressure returns to the basal level immediately after injection.

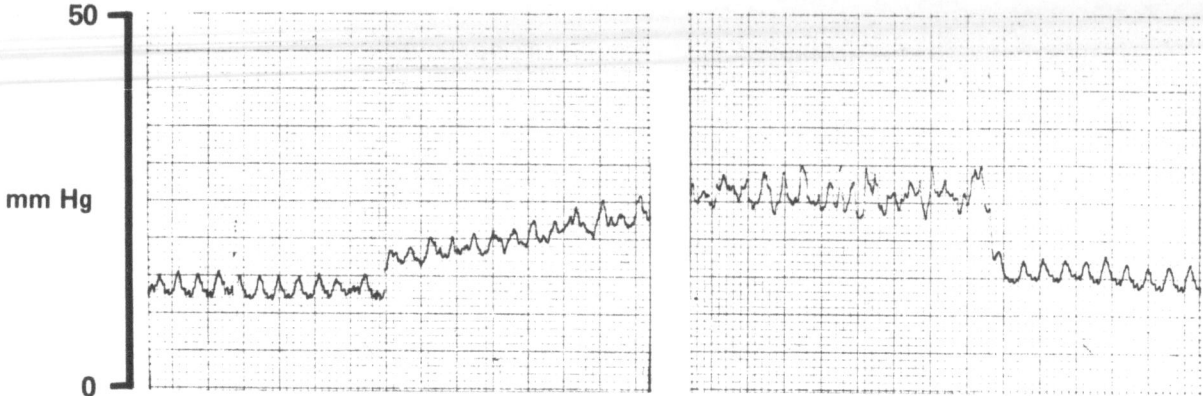

Fig. 6.3. Type II pressure filling curve is indicative of either spasm or organic obstruction (stenosis or calculi). The main features include a rising pressure during injection and a residual pressure (exceeding 2 mmHg) after injection. Functional spasm is diagnosed if the residual pressure after injection is abolished after the use of spasmolytic agents (CCK, ceruletide).

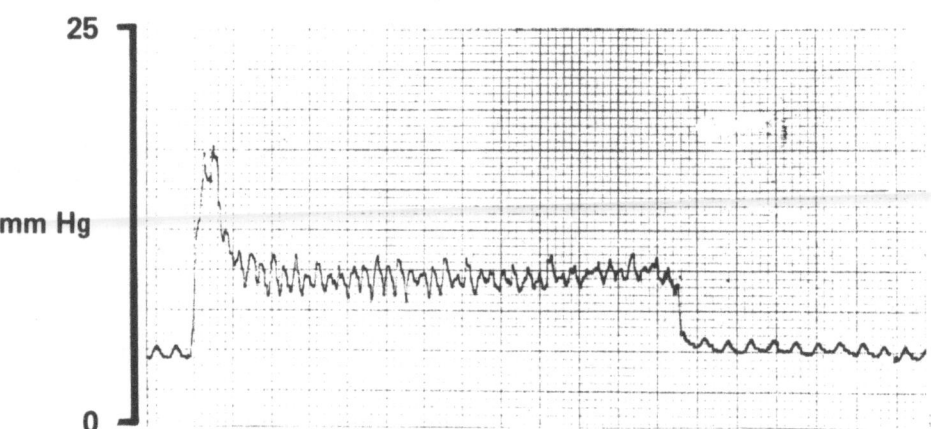

Fig. 6.4. Type III pressure filling curve. This indicates hypotonia of the SO and is encountered in 5–10% of patients with a normal operative cholangiogram.

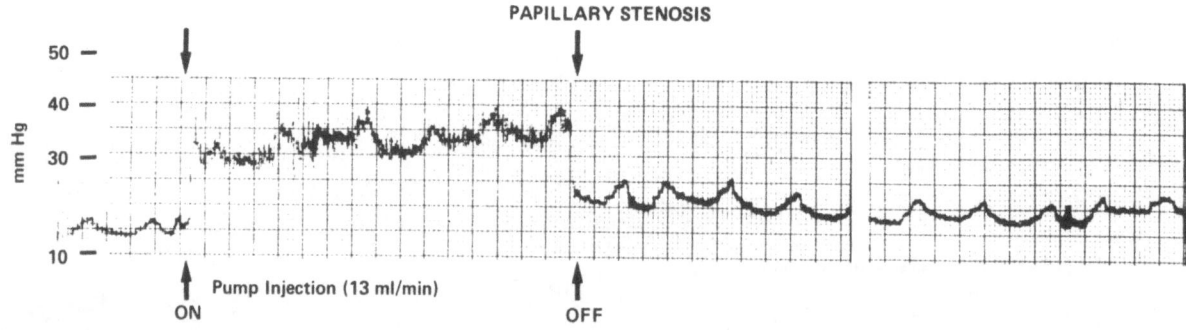

Fig. 6.5. Residual pressure after injection. The operative cholangiogram showed delayed emptying of contrast into the duodenum but no obvious stones. Common bile duct exploration identified 2 small calculi impacted in the common channel.

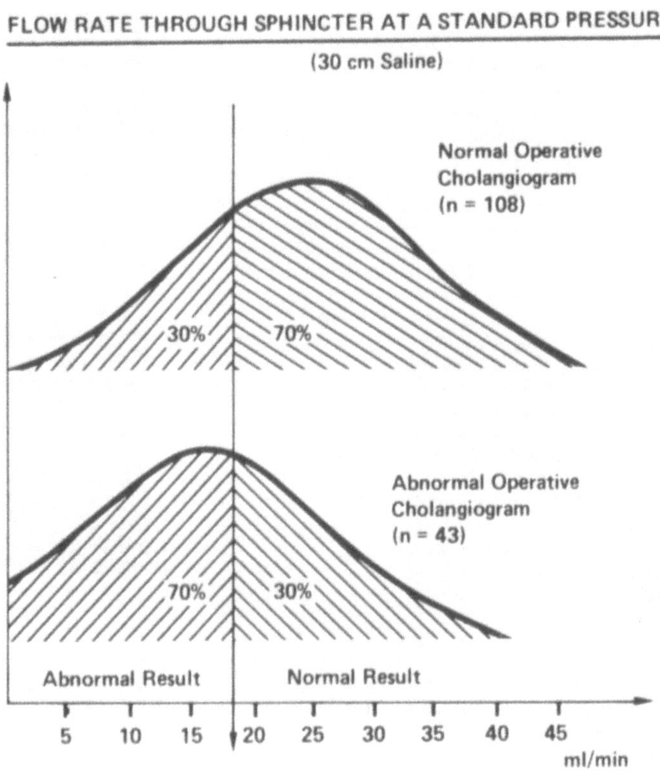

FLOW RATE THROUGH SPHINCTER AT A STANDARD PRESSURE HEAD

(30 cm Saline)

Normal Operative
Cholangiogram
(n = 108)

30% 70%

Abnormal Operative
Cholangiogram
(n = 43)

70% 30%

Abnormal Result   Normal Result

5   10   15   20   25   30   35   40   45

ml/min

Fig. 6.6. Values for flow rates through the SO in patients with a normal operative cholangiogram and in patients with ductal calculi. There is considerable overlap between the 2 populations such that debimetry is a poor prediction of ductal calculi.

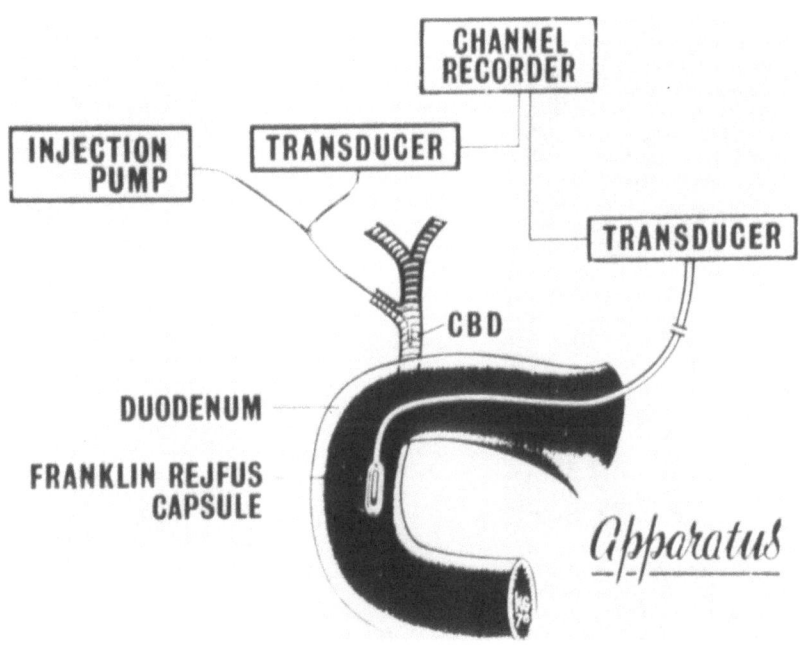

Fig. 6.7. Schematic representation of apparatus used by the author for operative cholangio-manometry.

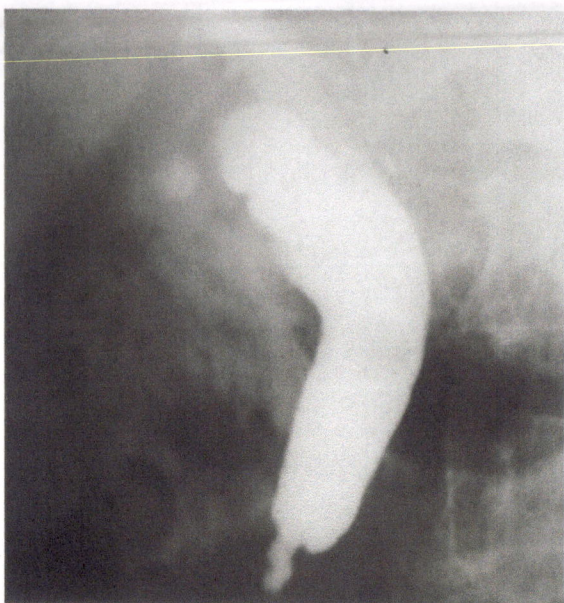

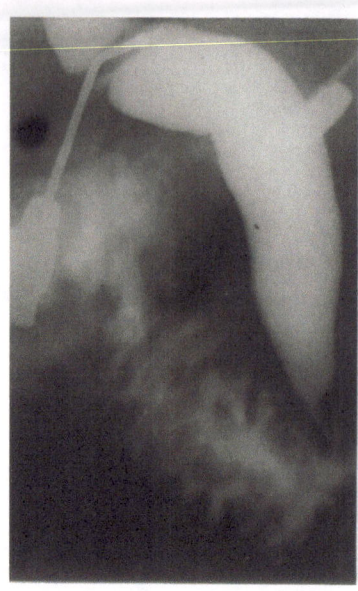

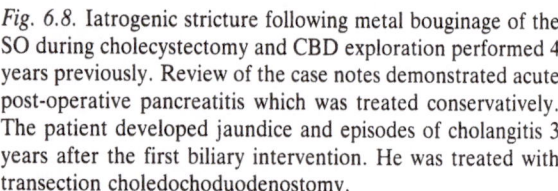

Fig. 6.8. Iatrogenic stricture following metal bouginage of the SO during cholecystectomy and CBD exploration performed 4 years previously. Review of the case notes demonstrated acute post-operative pancreatitis which was treated conservatively. The patient developed jaundice and episodes of cholangitis 3 years after the first biliary intervention. He was treated with transection choledochoduodenostomy.

Fig. 6.9. Contact selective cholangiogram showing stenosis of the SO with proximal bulbous distention of the infundibulum.

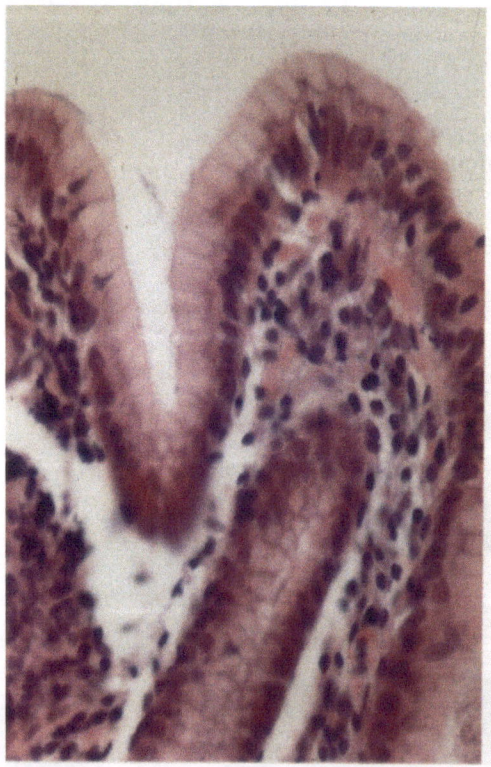

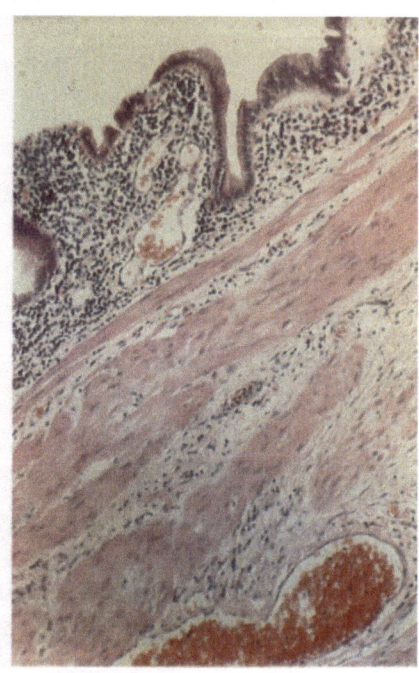

Fig. 6.10. (a) normal histology of a cholangioscopic biopsy from common channel. (b) histology of the common channel in a patient with papillary stenosis showing fibrosis, chronic cellular infiltrate and atrophy of the microvilli.

CHAPTER 7

EXPLORATION OF THE COMMON BILE DUCT

1. Introduction

Exploration of the common bile duct increases the morbidity and mortality in patients undergoing cholecystectomy. Most commonly it is performed to remove ductal calculi often in patients at risk because of jaundice and sepsis or both. Cholangitis may be present and the overall incidence of septicaemia in patients undergoing CBD exploration averages 10% (1). The reported mortality of choledochotomy is 3.5% (2). It is therefore imperative that the common bile duct is explored only when indicated. On the other hand the surgeon must avoid missing ductal pathology. In the past, surgeons adopted certain indications for exploration of the CBD such as multiple small faceted gallstones, history of jaundice, pancreatitis etc. Whilst these indications are still pertinent, the *decision to explore the CBD rests on the result of a properly conducted initial per-operative cholangiogram* (Chapter 4). There is one operative finding which always necessitates CBD exploration, i.e., palpable stone in a dilated CBD. It has been argued that in this instance per-operative initial cholangiography is superfluous and indeed may be technically unsatisfactory since the large volume of contrast needed to outline the biliary tract may obscure small calculi (3). This eventuality however is rare with graded injection and careful examination of the films at the early phase of contrast injection.

2. Technique of CBD exploration

The procedure entails the following steps:
1. Mobilization of duodenum and head of pancreas
2. Exposure of the CBD
3. Choledochotomy
4. Cholangioscopy
5. Additional procedures
6. Insertion of T-tube
7. Closure of choledochotomy
8. Completion cholangiography

2.1. Mobilization of duodenum and head of pancreas

This is an essential component of CBD exploration and is often overlooked. It is necessary for adequate palpation of the terminal bile duct and head of pancreas. It greatly facilitates cholangioscopic examination of the lower end of the CBD and ensures a tension free choledochoduodenostomy should this bilio-enteric anastomosis be deemed necessary by the surgeon.

The peritoneum is incised from the right extremity of the duodenal bulb alongside the 2nd part of the duodenum and then across to the left.

By means of careful pledge dissection the fibro-areolar tissue plane behind is opened allowing mobilization of the duodenal curve and head of the pancreas from the inferior vena cava and right renal vein (Fig. 7.1). At this stage the retro-duodenal end of the CBD is visualised prior to entering the pancreatic substance though occasionally it assumes a totally retro-pancreative course. The third part of the duodenum in next mobilised from the hepatic flexure and associated mesocolon until the uncinate process of the pancreas is displayed and in thin patients, the portal vein is seen. Thereafter thorough palpation of the terminal bile duct and head of pancreas is carried out (Fig. 7.2, Fig. 7.3).

2.2. Exposure of the CBD

The peritoneum overlying the extrahepatic bile duct is incised. It is important that undue mobilization of the peritoneum is avoided as this may impair the vascular blood supply to the CBD. The confluence of the cystic duct with the bile is displayed. Lymph node masses are present on the right edge of the retro-duodenal portion of the CBD. They are often found enlarged in secondary biliary intervention presumably from episodes of cholangitis. The bile duct wall itself is covered with a plexus of nerves and blood vessels. The latter are usually prominent and result in considerable oozing in secondary biliary interventions, particularly after episodes of bile duct obstruction and cholangitis. They are best dealt with by individual suture ligation with 4/0 black silk (Fig. 7.4).

2.3. Choledochotomy

Careful placing of the incision in the CBD is crucial. Fine (4/0) monofilament (prolene) stay sutures are inserted in either side of the midline 1.0 cm above the superior border of the duodenum (Fig. 7.5a, b). The incision is made with a sharp pointed scalpel and should not initially exceed 1.0 cm. A sucker is inserted close to the CBD before it is opened and a specimen of bile is obtained for culture. The choledochotomy wound is then held open by gentle traction on the stay sutures. Often in patients with ductal calculi, stones escape from the choledochotomy wound at this stage. Each stone is picked and laid on a swab. It is important that all the stones retrieved should at least equal the number seen on the initial cholangiographic films. Not infrequently however more stones are retrieved than indicated by the contrast films.

2.4. Cholangioscopy

This is dealt with in Chapter 5. It is our practice to perform an initial inspection of the extrahepatic biliary tract with the rigid endoscope and thereafter remove calculi or biopsy suspicious lesions under vision. When the cholangioscope is inserted, it is essential that the stay sutures are overlapped to approximate the edges of the choledochotomy around the endoscope.

2.5. Additional procedures

In centres where cholangioscopic facilities are not available, the surgeon often adopts other measures for stone removal. Dejardin's forceps are used to grasp loose stones. They are also used to crush stones impacted in the lower end of the CBD al-

though we do not advocate this technique since it has to be carried blind and may inflict trauma to the bile duct. To a large extent the use of biliary balloon catheters has replaced rigid blind instrumentation of the CBD for the removal of ductal calculi. They are however best used under cholangioscopic vision.

The procedure of blind bouginage of the lower end of the CBD with metal probes or dilators is still widely practised. It is a particularly dangerous procedure and should be avoided. The lower end of the CBD curves to the right before entry into the second part of the duodenum. Forcible blind probing of this delicate region often results in the formation of false passages, oedema, fibrosis and stricture (Fig. 7.6). The only instrument which can safely be passed through into the duodenum is a biliary balloon catheter. Some surgeons advocate inserting the rigid choledochoscope through into the duodenum. We consider this to be unnecessary and possibly traumatic. The best endoscopic assessment of the common channel is by careful inspection from above.

2.6. Insertion of T-tube

This is best discussed in relation to the findings on CBD exploration.

(a) Negative exploration. Overall this eventuality is encountered once in every 20 cases. It of course indicates faulty intra-operative decision making. However its occurrence cannot be completely avoided, though it can be minimized by good initial cholangiography and expert interpretation of films by a radiologist. The important practical point is to ensure without any doubt that there is indeed no intra-choledochal pathology and this can only be established with confidence by a properly conducted cholangioscopic inspection.

Controversy still exists as to whether a T-tube should be inserted in patients with negative CBD exploration. One study has suggested that T-tube drainage is associated with a higher incidence of wound infection and prolonged hospital stay (4). However, with the current practice of routine postoperative short term antibiotic prophylaxis (5, 6) this consideration does not apply. The disadvantages incurred by avoiding ductal drainage in these patients include, bile leakage from the choledochotomy wound and the inability to ascertain ductal clearance in the post-operative period without subjecting the patient to an ERCP.

An alternative compromise to this controversy which the author practises when he is confident that the exploration is indeed negative, after careful cholangioscopic inspection, is to insert a fine catheter into the CBD via the cystic duct and then close the choledochotomy incision. The catheter is held in place by a 2/0 catgut ligature to the cystic duct stump (Fig. 7.7).

It provides bile drainage and access for cholangiography in the post-operative period. The cannula is withdrawn 7 to 10 days after surgery.

(b) Positive exploration: The insertion of a T-tube of appropriate size and in the correct manner ensures safety and facilitates post-operative stone extraction via the T-tube tract in the eventuality of missed ductal calculi. It is imperative that the T-tube should not be smaller than size F16. The use of the Whelan Moss T-tube is considered preferable to the standard T-tube as it combines a wide long limb (F18–20) with a narrow intra-choledochal. limb. In order to ensure pliability and atraumatic removal, the horizontal limb of the T-tube should not exceed 2.0 cm in length. Various trimming techniques are used which ensure safe and easy withdrawal of the T-tube (Fig. 7.8). After insertion, the long limb is brought out at the distal extremity of the choledochotomy which is then closed above it. As indicated in chapter 8, the long limb of the T-tube should be exteriorized along a straight intra-abdominal course well into the right flank.

2.7. Closure of choledochotomy wound

This is effected by means of interrupted atraumatic fine sutures (Fig. 7.9). We prefer to use non-absorbable (prolene) suture material since this facilitates indentification of the bile duct should this be necessary at any subsequent surgical intervention and have not encountered any problems with stone formation provided the knots are tied on the outside. After flushing the system with 100 ml saline, a completion cholangiogram is performed.

3. Trans-duodenal exploration of CBD

This technique first described by Kocher (7) has

been advocated recently (8). It entails a preliminary duodenal mobilization followed by a duodenotomy. The sphincter of Oddi is then divided and Dejardin's forceps or a fibreoptic cholangioscope is introduced into the CBD (Fig. 7/10). The duct is then irrigated to clear any residual stones or mud. This approach has little to recommend it since it carries the following disadvantages:

1. Possible leakage from duodenotomy
2. Long term consequences of unnecessary sphincterotomy/sphincteroplasty
3. Risk of cholangitis
4. Acute haemorrhagic pancreatitis
5. Bleeding from the divided sphincter.

4. Intra-hepatic calculi

Multiple intrahepatic calculi are common in the Eastern hemisphere but fortunately rare in the West (9, 10). They may occur in an otherwise normal intrahepatic biliary tract or be associated with strictures, or cystic malformation (Caroli's disease). The vast majority are calcium bilirubinate stones. The surgical management varies with the exact pathology.

(i) *Removal via standard choledochotomy.* This is possible with loose stones in the major intrahepatic ducts by the use of the Berci-Shore choledochoscope. The author has successfully removed multiple intra-hepatic calculi in this way by using the instrument guide channel through which is inserted either a Dormia basket or biliary balloon catheter. Thorough irrigation to remove debris is necessary after evacuation of the stones. A T-tube is then inserted, the choledochotomy is closed and a completion cholangiogram performed.

(ii) *Extended choledochotomy.* This is practised as an alternative to the above. The incision in the bile duct is carried up to the region of bifurcation and the stones then cleared with scoopes, biliary balloon etc. Thorough irrigation is again necessary. Thereafter, closure of the choledochotomy, T-tube drainage and completion cholangiography are performed.

(iii) *Trans-hepatic lithotomy* – this is necessary for

stones impacted above a strictured intrahepatic duct. After localization of the affected duct, the hepatic substance is divided down to and including the duct. The stones are removed, the duct irrigated and the stricture then dilated. A silicone tube is the inserted into the intrahepatic duct beyond the stricture and the hepatic parenchyma sutured around it. Often this procedure is combined with CBD exploration with insertion of a second T-tube (Fig. 7.11, a, b, c).

(iv) *Hepatic resection.* This is reserved for cases with intrahepatic calculi involving the entire biliary ducts of one lobe.

It is our policy to perform a wide choledocho-duodenostomy in all these patients except those patients undergoing hepatic resection.

5. Assessment of terminal end of the CBD and sphincteric region

This is perhaps the most difficult area to assess intra-operatively and standard (panoramic) operative cholangiography may not provide sufficient information other than excluding calculi impacted in the lower end of the CBD. The techniques available to the surgeon with a special interest in disorders of sphincter function (stenosis, biliary dyskinesia) are:

1. Cholangioscopy and biopsy
2. Contact selective cholangiography (11)
3. Biliary manometry (Chapter 6)

The cholangioscopic appearances in patients with 'biliary dyskinesia' are normal as is the endoscopic biopsy of the common channel. The contact selective cholangiogram shows a dilated CBD with narrowing of the sphincteric region. Manometry shows a type II pressure filling curve with a residual pressure after injection which is abolished by CCK or ceruletide injection (Chapter 6).

The cholangioscopic appearances in benign papillary stenosis show distal cholangitis and debris with a rigid non-contractile common channel. The biopsy commonly demonstrate fibrosis with chronic inflammatory infiltrate.

The manometric findings are similar to those of biliary dyskinesia but are unaffected by spasmolytic agents. The findings on contact selective chol-

angiography are dilated CBD, smooth terminal stenosis, with alteration of the configuration of the infundibulum (trans-duodenal segment) which tends to display a bulbous dilatation. Periampullary diverticulae are often present but not invariable.

6. Post-operative removal of T-tube

This is normally removed on the 7th to the 10th day if the patient is progressing satisfactorily and the post-operative cholangiogram is unequivocally normal. It is our experience to perform a culture of T-tube bile before removal of the tube since in approximately 70% of patients with sterile bile at operation, bile culture becomes positive by the 4th–7th day with E. coli or Klebsiella organisms being the most commonly cultured species. This finding has been observed in other centres (12).

It seems likely that bacterial growth following common bile duct exploration and T-tube drainage may be a source of infection, prolonged morbidity and possibly of calcium bilirubinate stone formation. The latter may arise from deconjugation of bilirubin-glucuronide by baterial β-glucuronidase with the release of free bilirubin, the carboxyl group of which then combines with calcium to form insoluble calcium bilirubinate. A closed system of T-tube bile drainage minimizes secondary infection of bile postoperatively. It is our policy to administer appropriate antibiotics for 7–10 days if post-operative bile cultures are positive. There is however no indication to delay removal of the T-tube.

Indications for prolonged T-tube drainage. These are fairly clear cut. The T-tube should be left in situ:

(i) In all patients with missed ductal calculi shown on the postoperative cholangiogram. A period of 4 to 6 weeks is allowed to elapse for maturation of the T-tube tract before stone extraction via the T-tube tract with the flexible choledochoscope is performed. In the meantime the tube is spigoted and the patient can be discharged home but must be kept under periodic observation, and in any case should be advised to contact the surgeon immediately in the event of fever, rigors or jaundice.

(ii) Intraperitoneal leakage and peritonitis following withdrawal of the T-tube is a rare but serious complication. In the Cedars-Sinai experience it was observed in 5 out of 266 CBD explorations (1.8%) (13). This complication arises from inadequate maturation of the T-tube tract and is therefore encountered in the elderly, debilitated patients, after steroid or immunosuppressive/cytotoxic therapy and in patients with severe arteriosclerosis. It is recommended that the T-tube is clamped or spigoted on the 7-10 postoperative day but is left in situ for 3 weeks from the time of surgery. The T-tube is then withdrawn under fluoroscopic control. When the tube is 2/3 of the way out, contrast is injected through it into the tract. If leakage is observed, a guide wire is introduced into the CBD and a rubber catheter is inserted.

(iii) If the patient sustained operative injury of the bile duct and a primary repair was performed, the T-tube is left in situ as a stent for periods extending from 6 to 12 weeks.

7. Conclusion

Exploration of the CBD is a delicate procedure which should be approached with caution to minimize iatrogenic bile duct injury or missed pathology. Nowadays it involves a preliminary cholangiographic assessment on which is based the decision to explore the common duct. With the advent of cholangioscopy, intra-choledochal pathology can be visualized and blind instrumentation is avoided. A completion check with cholangioscopic inspection or T-tube cholangiography or preferably both is mandatory. The procedure therefore requires a planned approach without any short cuts. This will ensure safe biliary exploration and considerably minimize the incidence of complications including missed stones.

References

1. Engstrom J, Groth CG, Lundh G, Lonquist B: Infectious complications after surgery for biliary calculus. Acta Chir Scand 138:257–361, 1972.
2. Schein CJ, Shapiro N, Gliedman ML: Choledochoduodenostomy as an adjunct to choledocholithotomy. Surg Gynec Obstet 146:25–32, 1978.
3. Koch H, Stolte M, Walz V: Endoscopic lithotripsy in the common bile duct. Endoscopy 9:95–98, 1977.
4. Keighley MR, Burdon DW, Baddeley RM, et al: Complications of supraduodenal choledochotomy: A comparison of 3 methods of management. Br J Surg 63:754–758, 1976.
5. Strachan GJL, Black J, Powis SJA, et al: Prophylactic use of Cephazolin against wound sepsis after cholecystectomy. Br Med J 1:1254–1256, 1977.
6. Robson MC, Bogart JN, Heggers JP: An endogenous source for wound infections based on quantitative bacteriology of the biliary tract. Surgery 68:471–475, 1920.
7. Kocher T: Textbook of Operative Surgery, New York, MacMillan, 1965.
8. Carter AE: The transduodenal per-ampullary approach to common bile duct calculi. Ann Roy Coll Surg Eng 65:183–184, 1983.
9. Balasegaram M: Hepatic calculi. Ann Surg 175:149–154, 1972.
10. Sato T, Suzuki N, Takahashi W, Uematsu I: Surgical management of intrahepatic gallstones. Ann Surg 192:21–32, 1980.
11. Yvergneaux JP, Bauwens Ed, Van Outryve L, Yvergneaux Et: Benign stenosis of the papilla of Vater. Diagnoses of 119 cases with conventional and selective low radiomanometry. Acta Chir Belg 76:523–532, 1977.
12. Silen W, Wertheimer M, Kirshenbaum G: Baterial contamination of the biliary tree after choledochotomy. Am J Surg 135:325–327, 1978.
13. Berci G: Personal communication.

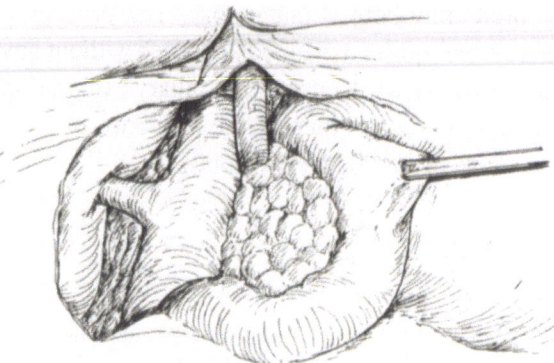

Fig. 7.1. Duodenal mobilization. The peritoneum is incised from the right extremity of the duodenal bulb alongside the 2nd part of the duodenum and then across to the left. The dissection is then carried out by gentle pledget dissection. The mobilization includes the 3rd part of the duodenum which is separated from the hepatic flexure and associated mesocolon.

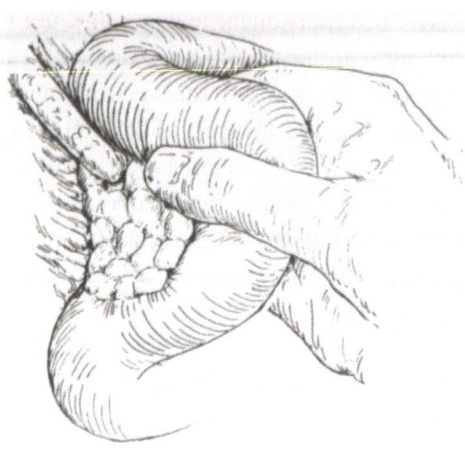

Fig. 7.2. The completed mobilization allows a careful and thorough palpation of the lower end of the CBD and the head of the pancreas.

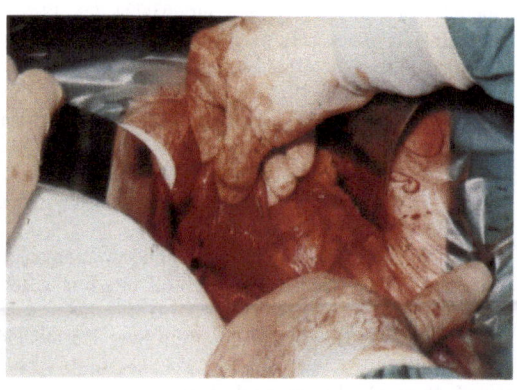

Fig. 7.3. Complete duodenal mobilization is essential for the performance of cholangioscopy and contact selective cholangiography.

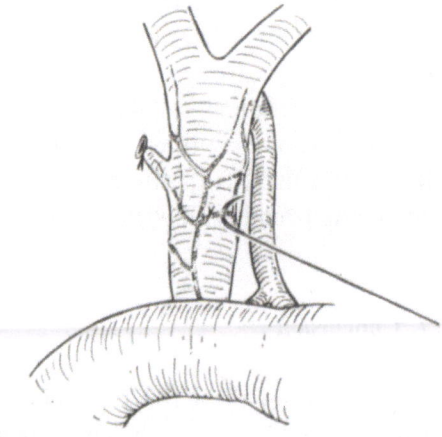

Fig. 7.4. Technique of individual suture ligation of pericholedochal veins during secondary biliary intervention using 5/0 atraumatic black silk sutures. Only those veins lying across the proposed choledochotomy site or those necessary for bile duct mobilization are suture ligated.

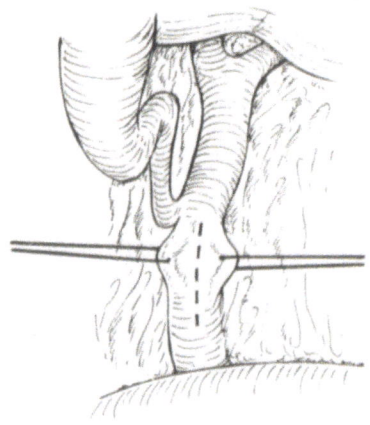

Fig. 7.5a. Diagramatic representation of the technique for CBD exploration. Fine monofilament sutures are used as stay sutures. The incision should not exceed 1 cm initially and is best sited in the supraduodenal region of the CBD about 1 cm proximal to the superior border of the duodenum.

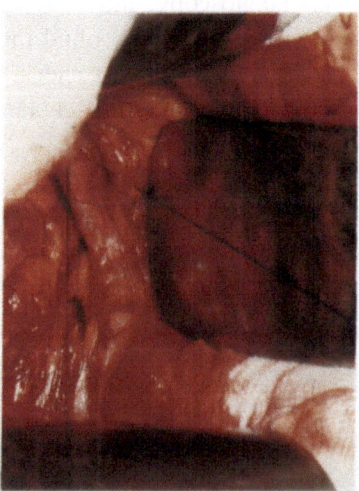

Fig. 7.5b. Operative demonstration of CBD exploration. Atraumatic prolene (5/0) has been for the stay sutures.

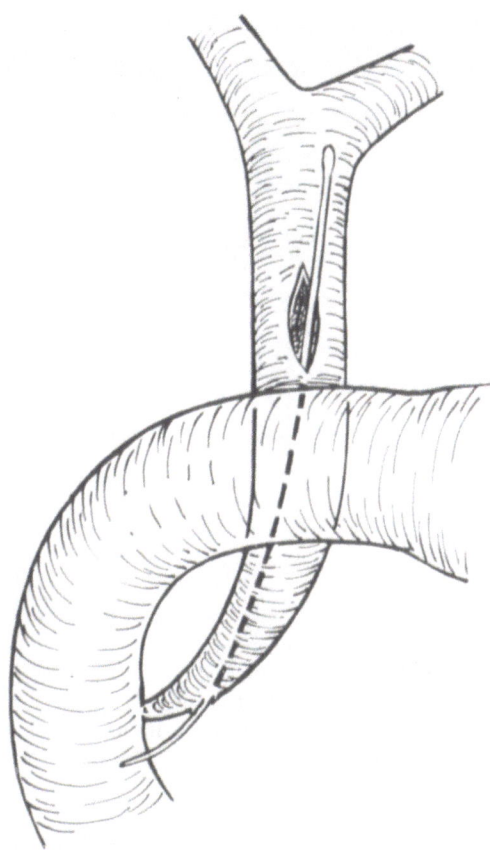

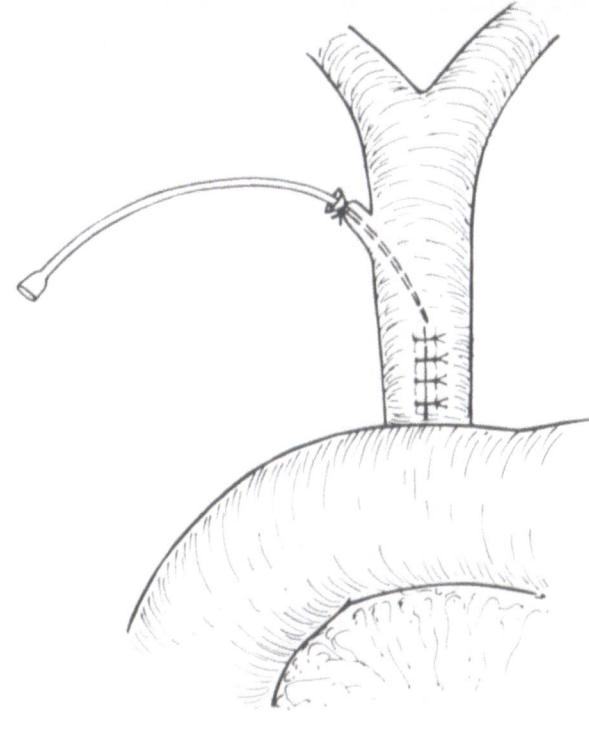

Fig. 7.6. The lower end of the CBD curves to the right before entering the duodenal wall. Blind probling with metal sounds may result in the creation of a false passage and traumatic damage. The long term consequences of this include cho-leduodenal fistula and stricture of the lower end of the CBD.

Fig. 7.7. Alternative to the use of T-tube in cases with *a negative CBD exploration.* A fine polyethylene cannula is inserted into the CBD and anchored to the cystic duct by a ligature. The choledochotomy wound is then closed. The cannula is sutured to the skin and connected to a closed bile drainage system. A post-operative cholangiogram can then be performed and the cannula removed on the 7th to 10th day. Removal is much easier than a T-tube and is not accompanied by any bile leakage.

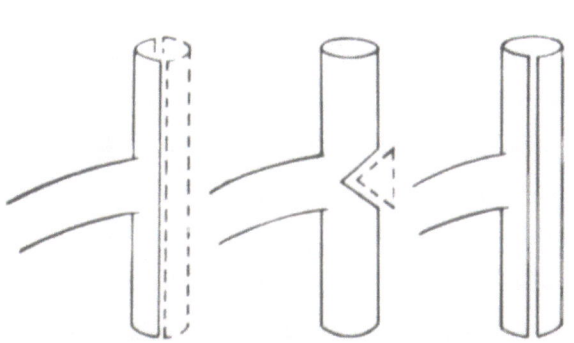

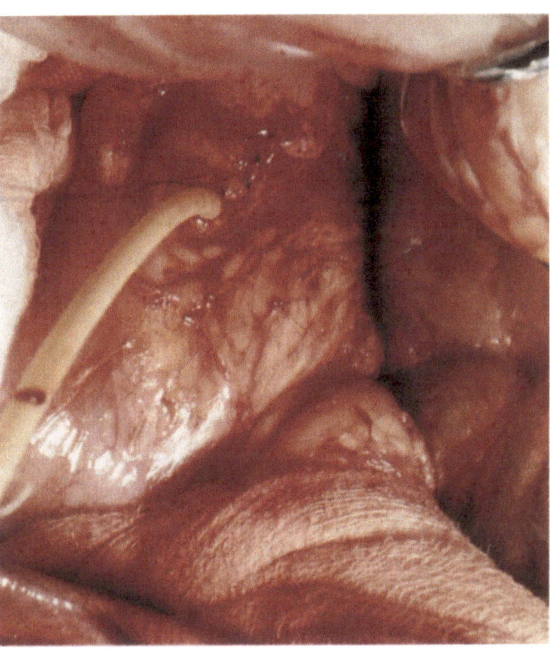

Fig. 7.8. Trimming techniques which facilitate the removal of the T-tube in the post-operative period. The horizontal limb should not exceed 2 cm in length.

Fig. 7.9. Closure of choledochotomy with interrupted 5/0 pro-lene sutures. The long limb of the T-tube emerges at the lower end of the choledochotomy wound.

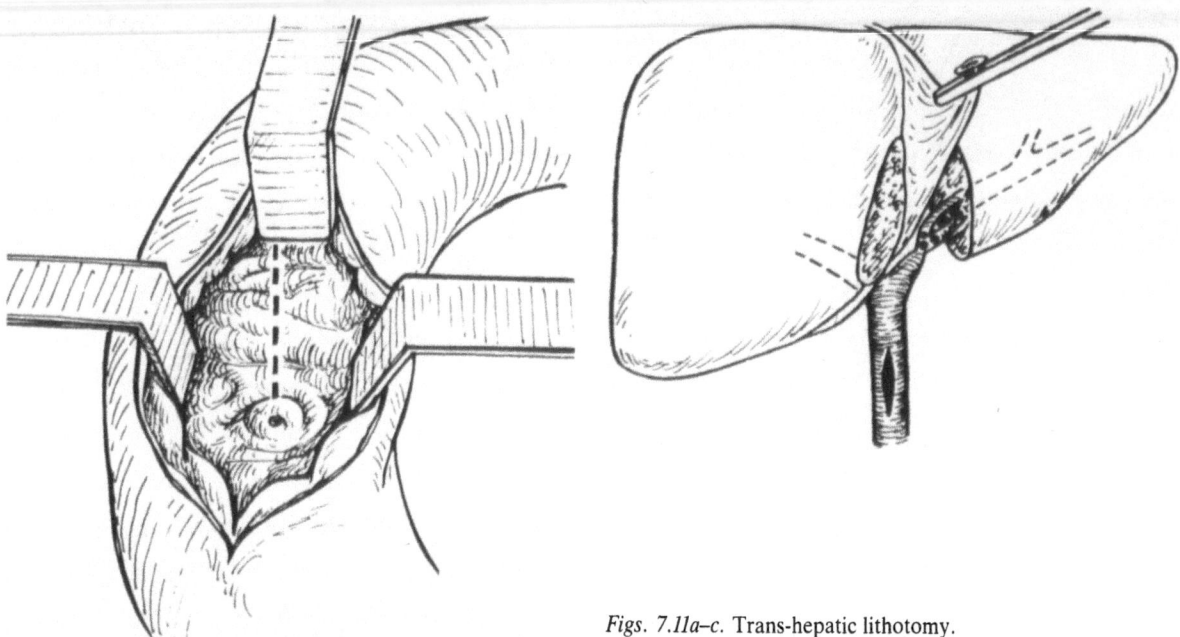

Fig. 7.10. Transduodenal exploration of the CBD. After the sphincterotomy, a Dejardin's forceps or a fibreoptic cholangioscope is introduced into the CBD.

Figs. 7.11a–c. Trans-hepatic lithotomy.

(a) After localization of the affected duct, the hepatic parenchyma is divided down to and including the duct. Often a stricture of the affected duct is encountered. In this eventuality a choledochotomy is performed.

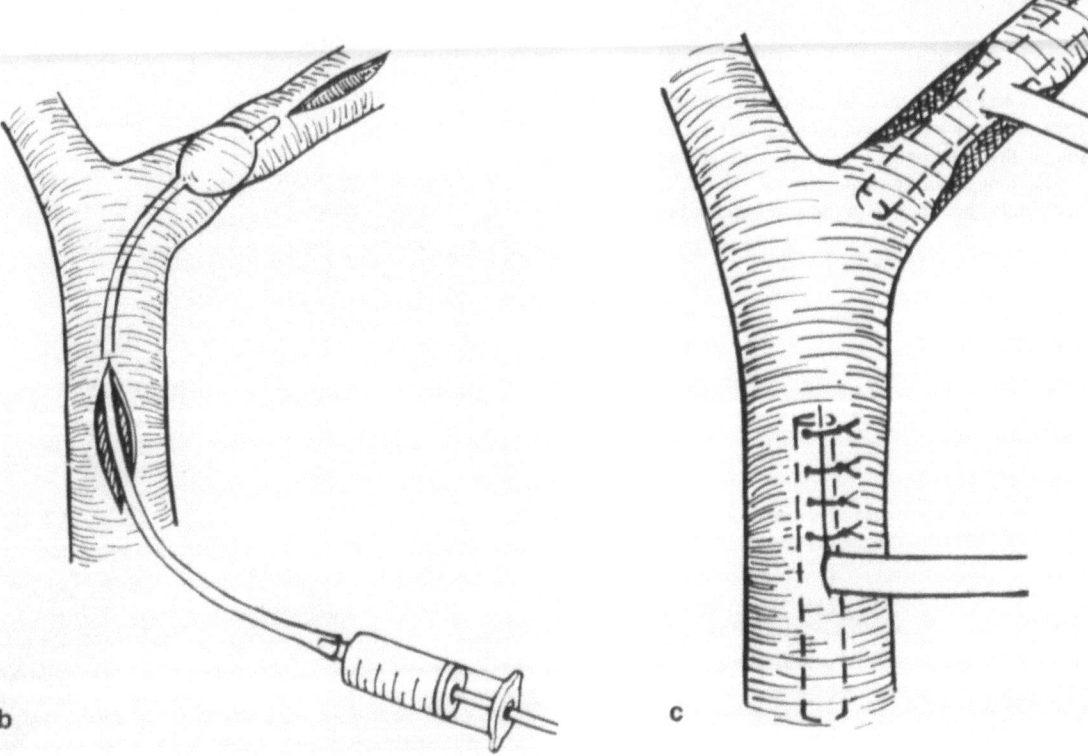

b

c

(b) The stricture is forcibly dilated by a balloon catheter introduced through the choledochotomy.

(c) A T-tube or silicone stent is then introduced into the affected intra-hepatic duct which is then irrigated thoroughly with heparinized saline. The hepatic parenchyma is then sutured around the stent. A second T-tube is then inserted into the CBD and the choledochotomy wound is closed.

CHAPTER 8

POSTOPERATIVE REMOVAL OF RETAINED STONES THROUGH THE T-TUBE TRACT
The combined fluorscopy-endoscopic technique

1. Introduction

Following choledocholithotomy missed calculi can be found in up to 10% of patients on the postoperative T-tube cholangiogram. These calculi may as yet be asymptomatic but some can signal their presence by increased output of bile from the T-tube, or the development of pain, fever, chills or jaundice.

When the retained calculus is small there is hope that it may pass spontaneously. The success of spontaneous passage, however, is unpredictable and cannot be relied upon. Apart from early sporadic reports of mechanical removal, the introduction of various agents through the T-tube has been advocated to reduce the size of the calculus (dissolution) and encourage its passage. Among these are heparin (1), chloroform (2), and sodium cholate (3). The effectiveness of these methods however has not been sufficiently great to warrant wide acceptance. More recently the use of mono-octinoin (Capmul) as a dissolving agent has gained support and has been shown to be effective in dissolving pure cholesterol stones. Since the calculus must be bathed by a relatively high concentration of the perfusate it is necessary to insert a small catheter with its tip near the calculus. It may be passed through the T-tube or percutaneously. Continuous perfusion for up to 7 to 10 days has been necessary and met with variable success (60–70%) (4, 5). During this period hospitalization is also required with frequent monitoring of hepatic function and re-checking of the catheter tip position by radiography.

2. Stone extraction via the T-tube

The simplest and safest way to handle this com-

plication is the mechanical extraction of the retained calculus which is discovered during postoperative T-tube cholangiography (6, 7, 8, 9, 10). The prerequisite of a successful removal is a relatively straight and wide tract (Figs. 8.1a–c).

Burhenne developed a steerable radio-opaque catheter which is introduced through the T-tube tract under fluoroscopic control (11, 12). A Dormia stone basket is advanced through this catheter to entrap or snare the stone(s) and withdraw it through the sinus tract (Figs. 8.2a–b). A drawback to this technique is the radiation exposure consequent on the fluoroscopy required to direct the manipulations. The calculi are often difficult to engage within the basket, particularly when the duct is curved and the operator has difficulty visualizing the thin wires of the basket on the television screen. Therefore, the fluoroscopic time will be prolonged. This results in excessive exposure to both patient and personnel. Stones located at the sphincter are difficult to engage and the basket may have to be passed repeatedly through the sphincter. This could inflict injury to the sphincter region, possibly resulting in stenosis.

3. Endoscopic method

Yamakawa converted Burhenne's technique to a direct endoscopic approach by introducing a flexible choledochofiberscope into the sinus tract to aid in the removal of retained stones under direct visual control (13, 14, 15). The size of this instrument (6.5 mm O.D.) and relative large turning radius caused some difficulty in negotiating the tract-CBD junction and produced patient discomfort or sharp pain because of stretching the duct. We employed, therefore, a smaller, more plaible, flexible bronchoscope which is only 4.8 mm in diameter and easier to maneuver within the duct. A Dormia basket, stone grasper, or balloon catheter (Fr. 4) can be introduced through the instrument channel. The actual entrapment and retrieval maneuver *is performed under direct visual control*. The sphincteric area can be well seen (16, 17). Subsequently, a smaller or more suitable fiberoptic choledochoscope became available and is now preferred* (Figs. 8.3a–c).

4. Preparation for stone extraction

Anticipating the possibility of a missed calculus and the necessity of a postoperative interventional procedure following CBD exploration, the surgeon should utilize a *large caliber T-tube*. The vertical limb should be brought out laterally to the flank in a relatively straight course perpendicular to the CBD and exiting through a *separate stab incision*. This facilitates passage of instruments through the tract in contrast to those cases wherein the tube is brought out anteriorly or takes a curved or looping course and enters the CBD at an acute angle.

After discovery of a retained stone on the T-tube cholangiogram performed approximately one week following surgery, we prefer to wait an additional five weeks before scheduling manipulation, in order to permit maturation of the T-tube tract. During this period most patients have their T-tube clamped but because of pain or cholangitis some may require continuous bile drainage. Each patient is seen in the fifth postoperative week at which time a bile sample is taken for culture and sensitivity. Appropriate antibiotics are started one day prior to the procedure and continued for three or four days post-manipulation.

The extraction is done on an outpatient basis except when severe underlying disease (cardiac or respiratory) necessitates precautionary hospitalization. The patient receives intravenous medication (Valium and Demerol) for sedation and analgesia during the extraction procedure. Hospitalized patients are sedated and monitored by an attending anesthesiologist.

5. Technique

The stone location is verified cholangiographically and a guide wire is introduced through the T-tube over which the T-tube is withdrawn. When the vertical limb of the T-tube is smaller than 16–18 Fr. or the size of the stone is too large, the tract is dilated by passing semi-flexible plastic dilating tubes over the guide wire into the CBD (Figs. 8.4a–b). We found the angioplasty balloon catheters very suitable and safe for dilatation of the tract.

After dilatation, the free end of the guide wire is inserted into the instrument channel of the fiberscope and under fluoroscopic control the scope is advanced over the guide wire into the CBD (Fig. 8.5). Further investigation and positioning of the scope is performed under *direct visual rather than fluoroscopic guidance*. Interrupted saline irrigation through the instrument channel clears any debris, permitting improved visualization of the lumen of the ductal system. When the stone is visualized, the stone basket is introduced through the instrument channel. By observing the wires of the open basket, appropriate maneuvers of the endoscope and the basket are *more rapidly and easily accomplished in order to entrap the calculus*. The procedure requires a team effort consisting of a radiologist and surgeon as well as trained technicians. Two hands are required to maneuver the endoscope while the second individual controls the stone basket. By coupling a teaching attachment to the eyepiece of the fiberscope, both operators have the advantage of directly viewing the movements of the introduced instruments within the CBD (Figs. 8.6a–f). Under direct observation, unnecessary passages through the sphincter are also avoided. If the wire basket cannot be advanced beyond the stone, a Fr. 4 arterial balloon catheter is employed to move the calculus. Care must be taken when inflating the balloon so that the duct is not overdistended. On occasion the stone can be wedged between the inflatable balloon of the catheter and the tip of the endoscope and successfully removed.

Following the procedure, a catheter is reintroduced into the extra-hepatic biliary system and secured by sutures at the skin level. Continuous bile drainage is maintained for a period of 24 h. Three or four days are allowed for clearing of debris induced by manipulation, prior to final chol-

---

* Manufacturer: Olympus Corp., Tokyo, Japan.

angiography. The catheter is then pulled after obtaining a negative cholangiogram.

6. Results

A successful stone extraction occurs in over 90% of those in whom it is attempted. Sixty-three patients were referred to us because of calculi found on the postoperative T-tube cholangiogram. Spontaneous passage had occured in four by the time we did our confirmation cholangiogram. In another patient the filling defect was removed and found to be a fibrin thrombus. This raised the possibility that some instances of 'spontaneous passage' may indeed be due to lysis of blood clots. In yet another patient a small papilloma was seen within the duct which was responsible for the radiolucent filling defect which suggested a calculus.

In the remaining 57 patients we were able to completely clear the duct of calculi in 54 cases (94.6%). In those patients for whom the procedure was unsuccessful either the T-tube inserted at surgery *was too small* (Fr. 8-10) or the tract *too tortuous*, thus preventing adequate dilatation and entry of instruments into the CBD. Twenty-eight patients required two or more sessions before we were able to declare the ductal system stone-free and finally remove the drainage tube.

7. Complications

In our series six patients developed fever which lasted for 24 to 48 h. Ten patients reported nausea or vomiting during the first 24 h following manipulation. Perforation of the T-tube tract occurred in two patients during dilatation of the tract and was verified by extravasation of injected contrast material. In both patients the extraction attempt was discontinued and we were able to reintroduce a guide wire back through the tract into the ductal system, over which a rubber catheter was advanced and continuous bile drainage was obtained. Both patients were hospitalized for observation for a period of 48 h and discharged without further complications. One patient's stone was extracted at a later stage while the other underwent CBD exploration.

Jaundice developed in one patient 18 months following manipulation and was found to be due to a stricture of the CBD at the sphincter. This stricture may have been the result of trauma sustained in this area during the repeated passages of instruments during the operation and manipulation in the postoperative period. A bilio-enteric bypass was performed in this case. *No mortality was encountered in this series*.

8. Discussion

If a retained stone is discovered in the postoperative period, the simplest and safest way to remove it is by way of the T-tube tract. *The success rate is predominantly influenced by the size and position of the T-tube* (Fig 8.7). Because of the difficulty in fluoroscopically assessing the position of the wires of the basket in relation to the calculus, using the Burhenne technique is often time-consuming and results in significant X-ray exposure to both patient and personnel. We employ a fiberoptic choledochoscope which is now available in a smaller and more suitable version. We have found the endoscopic approach to be faster, more precise and significantly reduces radiation exposure to both patient and personnel. The maneuvering of this scope in the CBD is well tolerated by patients and the stone manipulation is *performed under direct vision*. We do not extend the period of manipulation beyond 30 min during any one session. If the procedure is technically difficult we prefer to replace the drainage tube into the duct and recall the patient after one week for another session. Difficulty can occur if the calculus suddenly disappears into a long cystic duct stump (Figs. 8.8 and 8.9a–b). If it does not reappear soon, the patient is recalled a week later by which time the stone has hopefully migrated back into the CBD.

If the stone extraction efforts have failed and attempted dissolution has been unsuccessful, endoscopic sphincterotomy may be the next step. This technique requires a skilled endoscopist and hospitalization of the patient. Endoscopic sphincterotomy enjoys a success rate of approximately 80% but carries a morbidity rate of 10% and a mortality of 1% (18). In the event that all the above procedures fail to clear the ducts of calculi and the patient becomes symptomatic, re-exploration will be required.

In our series we achieved a success rate of 94.6% in removing retained stones through the T-tube tract by using a combined fluoroscopic-endoscopic approach. Among our patients there was minimal morbidity and no mortality.

References

1. Gardner B, Ostrowitz A, Masur R: Reappraisal of the possible role of heparin in solution of gallstones. Surgery 69:854–857, 1971.
2. Way LW, Motson RW: Dissolution of retained common duct stones. Arch Surg 10:99–119, 1976.
3. Pitt HA, Cameron JL: Sodium cholate dissolution of retained biliary stones. Mortality rate following intrahepatic infusion. Surgery 85:457–460, 1975.
4. Mack EA, Saito C, Goldfarb S, Crummy AB, Thistle JL, Carson GL, Babayan VK, Hoffman AF: A new agent for gallstone dissolution. Surg Forum 24:438–438, 1978.
5. Mack E, Patzer EM, Crummy AB, Hofman AF, Babayan VK: Retained biliary tract stones. Arch Surg 116:341–344, 1981.
6. Bean WJ, Mahorner HR: Removal of residual biliary stones through the T-tube tract. S Med J 65:377–378, 1972.
7. Bean WJ, Smith SL, Calonje MA: Percutaneous removal of residual biliary stones. Radiology 113:1–9, 1974.
8. Mazzariello R: Removal of residual biliary tract calculi. Lancet 1:1044–1045, 1971.
9. Mondet A: Tecnica de la extraccion incruenta des los calculos en la lithiasis residual del coledoco. Bol Soc Cir Buenos Aires, 46:278–290, 1972.
10. Mazzariello R: Review of 220 cases of residual biliary tract calculi treated without re-operation. Surgery 73:299–306, 1973.
11. Burhenne JJ: Nonoperative retained biliary tract stone extraction. Am J Roentgenol 117:388–399, 1973.
12. Burhenne JJ: Complications of non-operative extraction of retained common duct stones. Am J Surg 131:260–262, 1976.
13. Yamakawa T: An improved choledocho-fiberscope and non-surgical removal of retained biliary calculi under direct visual control. Gastrointest Endoscop, 22:160–165, 1976.
14. Moss JP, Whelan JG, Powell HW, Dedman T, Oliver WJ: Post-operative choledochoscopy via the T-tube tract. JAMA 236:2781–2782, 1976.
15. Berci G, Hamlin JA: A combined fluoroscopic and endoscopic approach for retrieval of retained stones through the T-tube tract. Surg Gynec & Obstet 153:237–240, 1981.
16. Berci G, Hamlin JA: Retrieval of retained stones. In: Operative Biliary Radiology. Berci G, Hamlin JA (eds), Baltimore, Williams & Wilkins, 1981, p 147–158.
17. Chen MF, Chou FF, Wang CS, Jang YI: Experience with and complications of postoperative choledochofiberscopy for retained biliary stones. Acta Chir Scand, 148:503–509, 1982.
18. Berci G: Endoscopic retrograde sphincterotomy. In: Current Gastroenterology and Hepatology. Gitnick (ed). Boston, Houghton-Mifflin 1979.

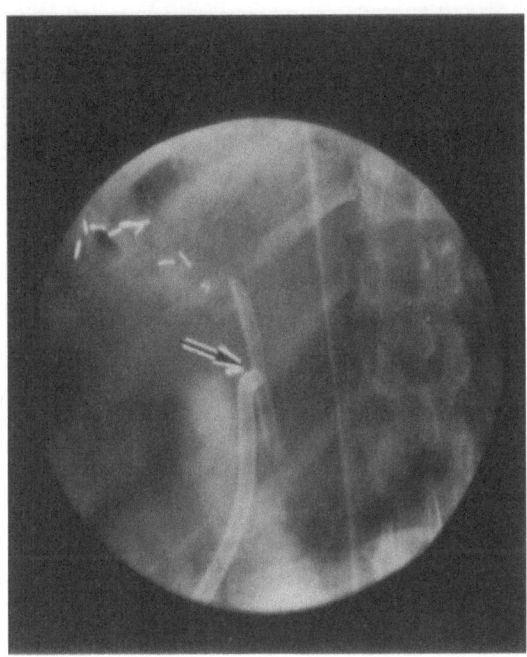

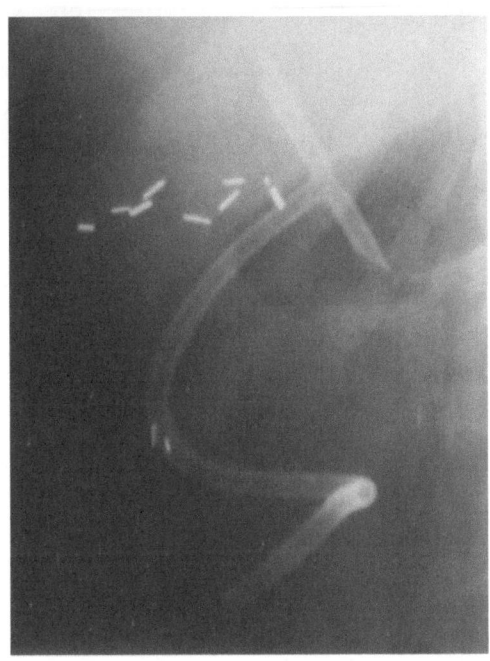

Fig. 8.1a. Angulated vertical limb near the CBD (arrow). The horizontal limbs should be kept relatively short.

Fig. 8.1b. 'S' shaped curve of the vertical limb.

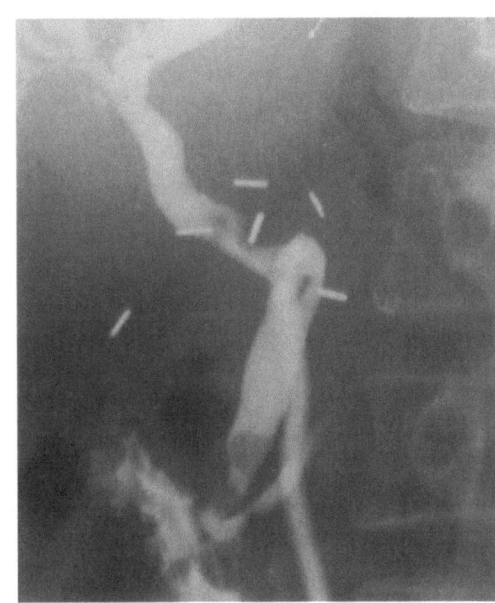

Figs. 8.1a–c. The prerequisite of a successful stone removal via the T-tube tract is a relatively large and straight sinus. This can be achieved if the surgeon is aware of the importance of this aspect. Examples of poorly placed T-tubes.

Fig. 8.1c. This small (Fr. 14) T-tube was brought out in the mid-line with a sharp curvature.

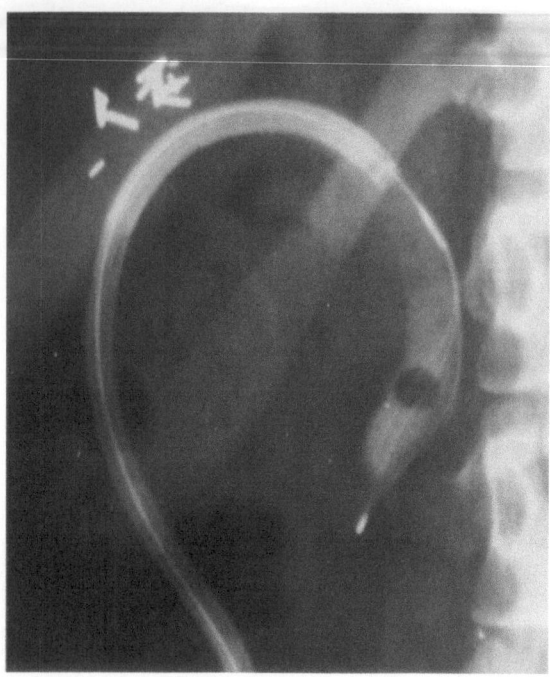

Fig. 8.2a. With the CBD opacified to localize the stone, the steerable catheter and stone basket are introduced. The basket wires which are well seen on the radiograph are often difficult to identify fluoroscopically because of the diminished resolving capacity of the television. It may, therefore, be necessary to make multiple passes by the stone with the basket before a successful entrapment.

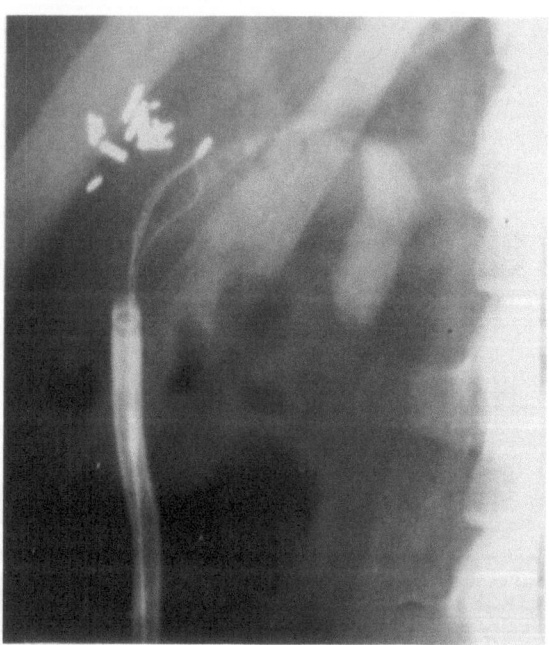

Fig. 8.2b. The stone is withdrawn into the tract. If the CBD-tract junction is acutely angulated or the stone is not in the appropriate position in the semi-closed basket it can be lost during withdrawal.

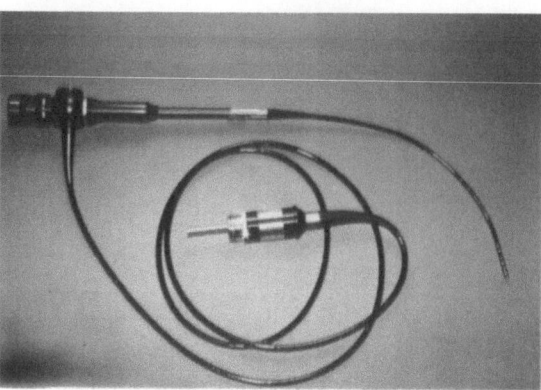

Fig. 8.3a. The flexible fiberoptic choledochoscope (O.D. 4.8 mm) with one instrument channel.

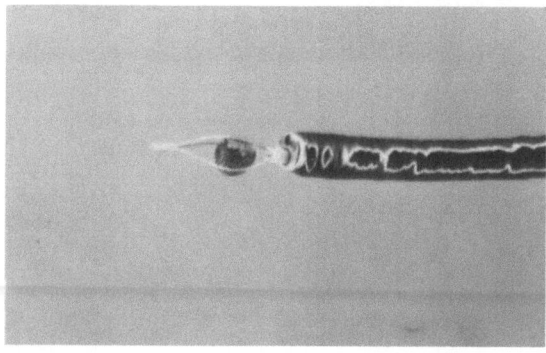

Fig. 8.3b. The great impact of endoscopic stone removal is the entrapping of a stone under visual control. It is much more precise and faster than using fluoroscopic technique alone.

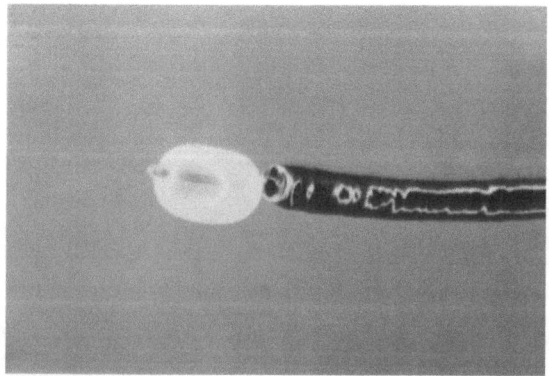

Fig. 8.3c. A Fr. 4 balloon catheter can be advanced beyond the stone and inflated. The stone can be moved or occasionally wedged between the balloon and the tip of the scope and withdrawn.

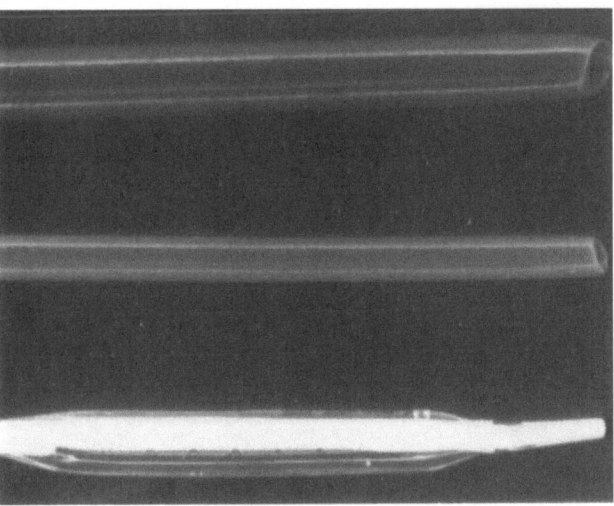

Fig. 8.4a. Top: Semi-flexible plastic dilators of various sizes. *Bottom:* Balloon catheter (Grundzig type) which is ideally suited for dilatation.

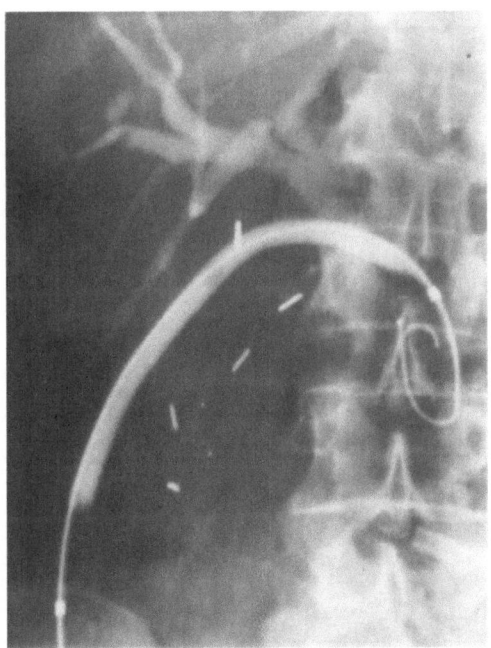

Fig. 8.4b. A 10 cm balloon catheter is introduced over the guide wire and distended with contrast material. The entire tract can be dilated in one session.

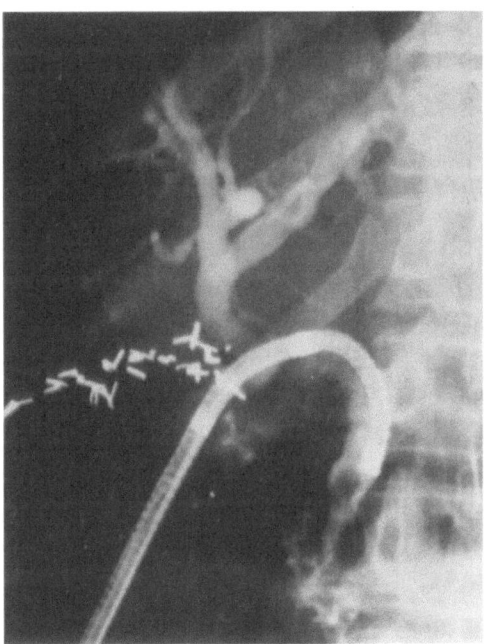

Fig. 8.5. Scope introduced into the distal duct. If difficulties occur during introduction, contrast material can be injected through the instrument channel and the anatomy outlined. Stone in front of the tip of the scope.

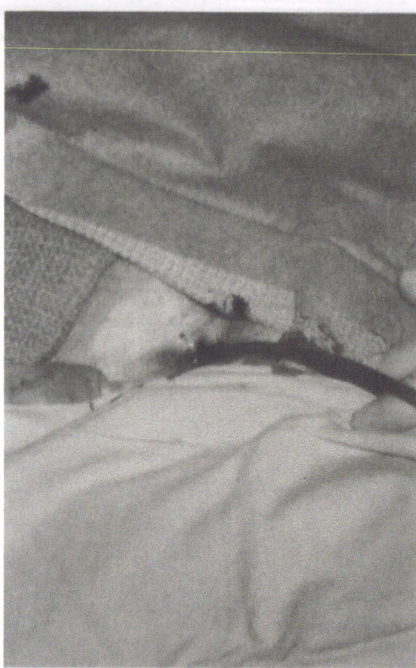

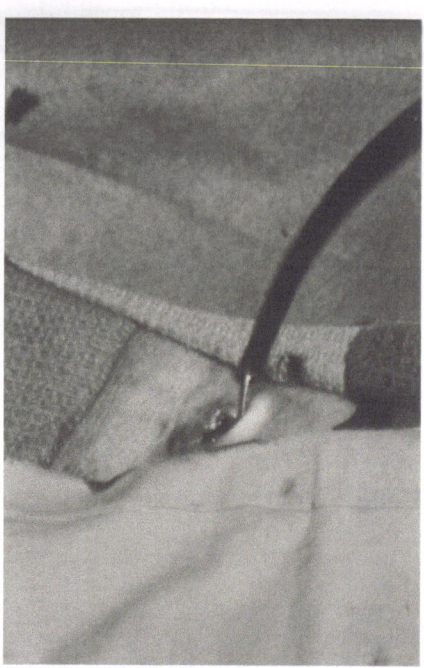

Fig. 8.6b. The scope is introduced under fluoroscopic control to the sinus tract-CBD junction. At this point the guide wire is removed and the instrument is advanced under direct vision. If required, contrast material can be injected through the instrument channel to outline the anatomy for fluoroscopic observation.

Fig. 8.6a. After dilatation the flexible instrument is advanced over the guide wire.

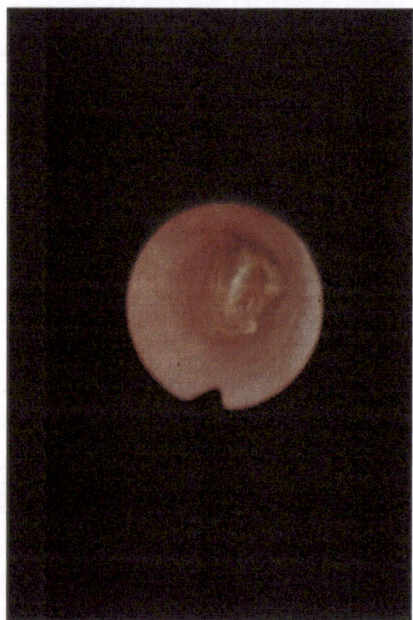

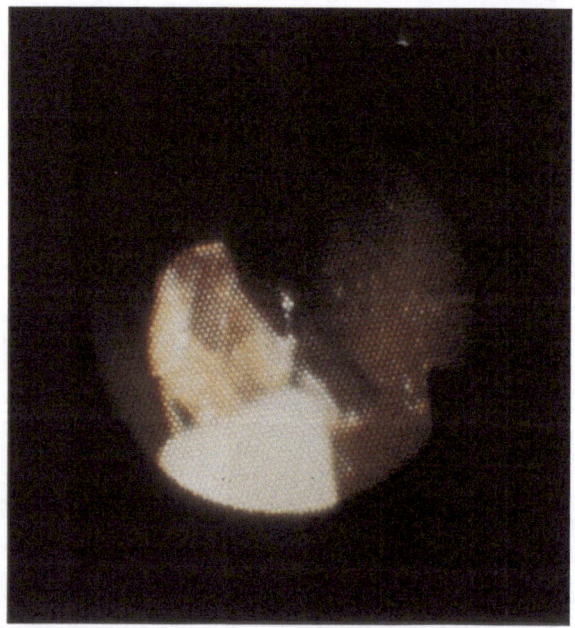

Fig. 8.6c. The distal (impacted) stone is well seen. The position of the basket or balloon can be changed according to need and anatomy without *unnecessary* passage of the instrument through the sphincter.

Fig. 8.6d. Basket entrapping a stone as seen through the flexible endoscope.

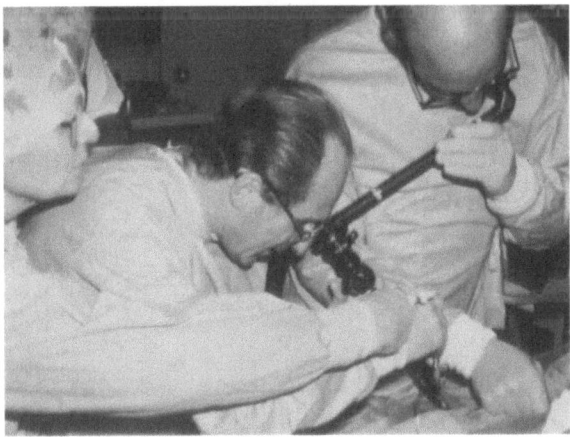

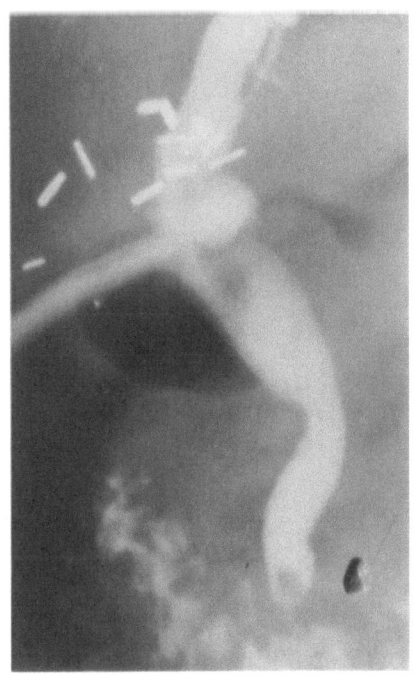

Fig. 8.6e. Teamwork is required for endoscopic stone retrieval. Instrument control requires two hands while a second individual maneuvers the stone basket. A nurse is often necessary to supply an extra hand in the procedure. Due to respirations or movements of a smaller stone, all maneuvers have to be precisely coordinated.

Fig. 8.6f. Cholangiogram demonstrating an impacted stone. Photograph of the extracted stone beside.

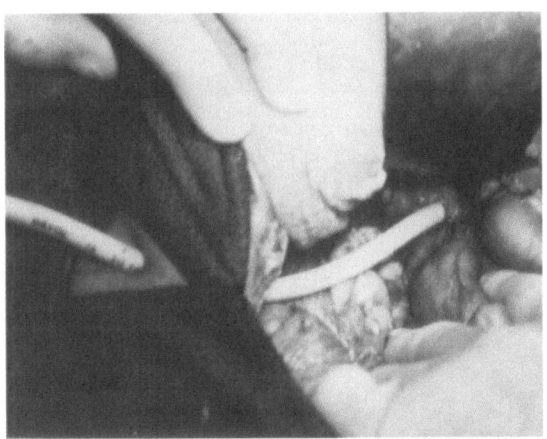

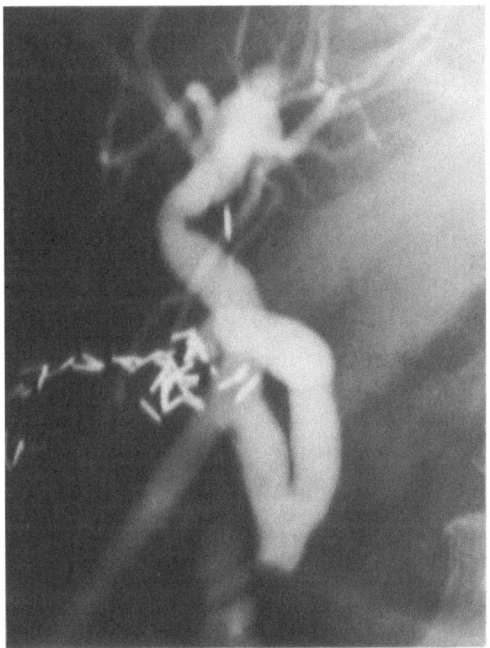

Fig. 8.7. The ease with which a successful extraction is accomplished is related to the size and course of the sinus tract. The T-tube should be brought out in the flank, if possible without loops or kinks. The recommended minimum size of the vertical limb is Fr. 16.

Fig. 8.8. A retained stone in the ampulla with a long dilated cystic duct stump. During manipulation the stone can easily disappear in this hiding place. (For details see text).

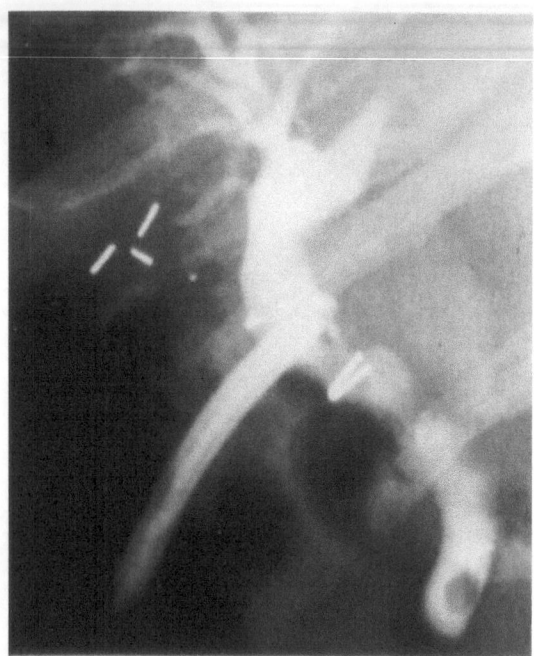

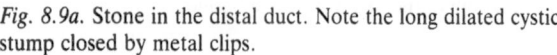

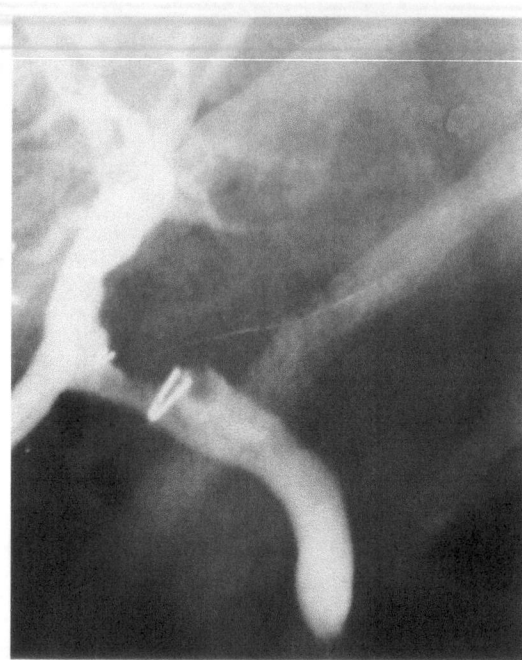

Fig. 8.9b. Same patient as shown in Figure 8.8a but the calculus moved into the cystic stump (hiding place) during manipulation. The patient was sent home and recalled one week later when the stone was again within the CBD and the removal attempt was successful.

Fig. 8.9a. Stone in the distal duct. Note the long dilated cystic stump closed by metal clips.

SUBJECT INDEX

A

Aberrant ducts, 24
Abnormal circulating anticoagulants, 8
Accessoires, 55
Adrenalin, 72
Advantages, 30
Aerobic gram-negative, 3
After biliary surgery, 7
Ampulla, 57
Ampullary stenosis, 58
Amylnitrite, 72
Anaerobic infections, 3
Angioplasty balloon catheter, 90
Anomalies of surgical importance, 24
Anterograde, 10
Antibiotic regimes, 8
Assessment of terminal end of the CBD and sphincteric
    region, 84
Atropine, 72
Attachable stone forceps, 56

B

Bacteremia, 28
Balloon catheter, 55, 56
Benign papillary stenosis, 84
Berci-Shore, 74
Bifurcation, 56
Bile duct rupture, 28
Biliary balloon catheter, 55, 82
Biliary dyskinesia, 84
Biliary pressure indices, 72
Blind bouginage, 82

C

Caerulein, 72
Calculi, 57
Cannula, 74
Cannulation techniques, 20
Caroli's disease, 83
Caroli's instrument, 73
Chloroform, 80
Cholangioscopy, 55, 82
Cholangitis, 7, 57
Cholecystectomy, 10
Cholecysto-Cholangiogram, 25
Cholecystokinin (CCK), 71
Choledocholithiasis, 57, 58
Choledochotomy, 82
Choledochotomy incision, 56
Clotting factors concentrates, 8
Common bile duct explorations, 20
Completion cholangiogram, 21
Completion cholangiography, 30

Complications, 59, 91
    after biliary surgery, 7
    of T-tube removal, 28
Contrast material, 22
Cystic artery, 10
Cystic duct, 10, 25
Cystic duct remnant, 25, 57

D

Debimetry, 71
Dejardin's forceps, 82
Diagnostic accuracy, 30
Disadvantages, 30
Disc to the eyepiece, 56
Disorders of the sphincter of Oddi, 74
Dissolving agent, 89
Dormia stone basket, 55, 56
Drainage, 11
Drainage of cystic duct in the right hepatic duct, 24
Ductal diverticula and choledochocele, 24
Dynamic (transducer) manometry, 73

E

Endoprosthesis,
    endoscopic, 9
    percutaneous transhepatic, 9
Endoscopic appearance, 56
Endoscopic method, 89
Endoscopic papillotomy, 9
Endoscopic sphincter zone activity, 73
Epsilon Aminocaproic Acid (AECA), 8
Equipment, 21
Excessive injection, 28
Exploration of the common bile duct, 81
Exposure of the CBD, 81
Extended choledochotomy, 83

F

Fenwal pressure irrigation system, 56
Fibrinogen degradation producers (FDP), 8
Fibrinolytic state, 8
Filling pressure curves, 72
Flow rate (debimetry), 73
Fluoro-cholangiographic technique, 23
Fewh frozen plasma, 8
Functional disorders, 75
Functional obstruction (spasm), 75

G

Gastrin, 71
General complications, 7
Glucagon, 71
Glyceryl nitrite, 72

Gravimetric (hydrostatic) techniques, 73
Grid, 21

H
Haemorrhagic complications, 8
Heparin, 89
Hepatic resection, 84
High risk factors, 3
Hypotomic sphincter, 76

I
Iatrogenic bile duct injury, 3
Iatrogenic stricture, 74
Illumination, 10
Impaire platelet function, 8
Incision
    Kocher's, 9
    Mayo Robson, 9
    midline, 9
    right paramedian, 9
    transverse, 9
Incremental pressure and recovery time, 73
Induction of diuresis, 9
Infectious complications, 3, 7
Initial and/of completion cholangiograms, 20
Initial cholangiography, 30
Injected volume, 22
Insertion of T-tube, 82
Instrumentation, 55
Intra-abdominal sepsis, 7
Intra-hepatic calculi, 83
Intramuscular vitamin K analogue, 8
Intraoperative cholangiography, 19
Isoproterinol, 72

M
Maintenance, 59
Malabsorption of vitamin K, 8
Manometry, 71
Mecholyl, 72
Mobilization
    of duodenum, 56, 81
    of head of pancreas, 81
Mono-octinoin, 89
Morphine, 72

N
Negative exploration, 82
Neoplasms, 58
Normal findings, 57

O
Oral administration of bile salts, 9
Osmotic (mannitol) diuretic, 9
Overhead lighting, 10

P
Papillary stenosis (choledocho-duodenal junctional stonisis), 75
Papillitis/oedema, 74
Passage (yield, opening) pressure, 72
Pathophysiology, 8
Patient's positioning, 20
Pethidine, 72
Pharmacological agents, 72
Phenylephrine, 72

Platelet transfusions, 8
Positive exploration, 83
Postoperative bronchopneumonia, 7
Pre-operative decompression
    percutaneous transhepatic, 9
    trans-cystic, 9
Pre-operative hydration, 9
Preparation for stone extraction, 90
Prophylactic antibiotic treatment, 8
Prophylactic short term antibiotic therapy, 3
Prothrombin time, 8

R
Radiation protection, 25
Reformed calculi, 28
Removal of T-tube, 84
Renal failure, 8
Residual pressure, 73
Resting (initial, interdigestive) pressure, 72
Results, 91
    of operative cholangiography, 30
Retained calculus, 89
Retrograde, 10

S
Scope, 60 mm, 55
Scopolamine, 72
Scout film, 21
Secretin, 72
Semi-flexible plastic dilating, 90
Septicaemia, 7
Short cystic duct, 24
Sodium cholate, 83
Spasm, 72
Sphincter, 57
    of Oddi motor activity, 75
Spiral cystic ducts, 25
Standard choledochotomy, 83
Standard 40 mm horizontal, 55
Stay sutures, 56
Steerable radio-opaque catheter, 89
Sterilization
    autoclaving, 59
    gas, 59
Stone extraction via the T-tube, 89
Suction trocar cannula (Mayo Oschner), 10
Surgical light, 10
Syrringe barral technique, 73

T
Technique, 21, 56, 81, 90
    of operative biliary manometry, 73
Trans-duodenal exploration of CBD, 83
Trans-hepatic lithotomy, 83
T-tube cholangiogram, 60

U
Unsuspected stones, 20
Usage, 71

V
Vitamin K dependent factors, 8

W
Whelan Moss T-tube, 83